Brigid McConville is
ising in health and so
national newspapers magazines including the *Daily Telegraph*, *Daily Mail*, *Independent*, *The Times*, *Guardian*, *Marie Claire*, *SHE*, *Woman* and *CHIC*. Her books include *Women Under the Influence: Alcohol and Its Impact* (Pandora) and *Mixed Messages: Our Breasts in Our Lives* (Penguin).

She lives in Somerset with her partner John and their children Maeve, Arthur and Rory.

Jonathan Pugh is a highly successful cartoonist whose work appears daily in *The Times* and regularly in the London *Evening Standard*. He has also illustrated a number of books.

Also by Brigid McConville

Women Under the Influence: Alcohol and Its Impact
Mixed Messages: Our Breasts in Our Lives

COMING UP FOR AIR

Self help for asthma sufferers

Brigid McConville

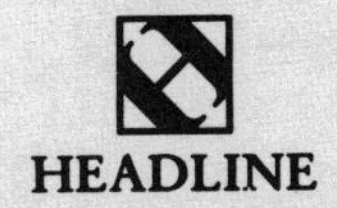

HEADLINE

First published in 1995
by HEADLINE BOOK PUBLISHING

10 9 8 7 6 5 4 3 2 1

ISBN 0 7472 4387 5

Typeset by
Letterpart Limited, Reigate, Surrey

Printed and bound in Great Britain by
Cox & Wyman Ltd, Reading, Berks

HEADLINE BOOK PUBLISHING
A division of Hodder Headline PLC
338 Euston Road
London NW1 3BH

For Rory, with love.

Acknowledgements

Special thanks to all those – young people, parents, children and grandparents – who gave their time to tell me about the impact of asthma on their lives. Margaret Williams, Madeleine Morey, Edward Willis, Lucy Willis, Tanza Tottle, Sally Tottle, and Beryl McConville are among those who have particularly helped with ideas and comments.

The National Asthma Campaign – both at head office and through their volunteers – have contributed generously of their knowledge and information and have double-checked my manuscript for accuracy. Dr Martyn Partridge and Dr Jill Warner, experts in their field, have given me valuable pointers while Edwina Currie, Niamh Cusack and Rory O'Neill have also given of their time and experience.

I am indebted, too, to Dr Rajendra Sharma, Medical Director of 101 Clinic and The Good Health Company, for kindly offering to check my manuscript.

Contents

CHAPTER 1

The Experience of Asthma

JANET'S STORY

'I've done the London to Brighton bike race on a tandem!' Janet tells me as we chat on the phone. Now to complete that fifty-mile ride over hill and dale is quite an achievement for anyone, but for a forty-two-year-old who suffers from asthma, it has a very special significance.

It means that Janet has taken charge of her own health and is now firmly in control of her asthma, which not long ago was disrupting – and even threatening – her daily life: 'There was a time when I simply wasn't facing up to the disease; I was denying it. I felt quite bitter about it: it seemed so unfair. Why should I have this disease? It was an encumbrance and I wanted to get on with my life.' Understandable as these feelings are, they left Janet vulnerable to becoming ill, so that when she had a serious asthma attack, she found that her life was suddenly on the line.

'I'd had a bad attack and was going blue,' she tells me. 'Fortunately, my husband took me to the nearest casualty department, rather than my usual hospital – the London – which was a few miles further away. My doctor later told me that I was unlikely to have survived the further distance.'

That experience changed Janet's attitude dramatically. 'I

now respect the disease,' she says, 'and I can face it. I have confidence in taking it on and I don't feel at its mercy.'

Since then Janet has been taking very good care of herself, using a self-management plan which she has worked out with her GP. 'In the past I felt powerless to intervene in my asthma,' she says. 'But now I know that there are steps I can take – quite clear steps – which will stop me from going down that slippery slope. I know where I'm going and it suits me wonderfully!'

And although it may sound strange at first, Janet feels that her asthma – or at least her battle to win control of it – has changed her life for the better: 'I wouldn't be the person that I am if I hadn't had asthma,' she says thoughtfully. 'It has made me very self-reliant and, I hope, sensitive. I've had too many bad times not to really appreciate life.'

If, like Janet, you have suffered from the distressing and sometimes frightening symptoms of asthma, or if your child has developed asthma, you will also know that this is a very complex condition. It not only has a wide range of potential causes and 'triggers', but there are many kinds of medicine to hold it in check, too.

Like Janet, you may have despaired at times of ever finding a way through the maze of symptoms and medicines to the level of treatment – self-help or orthodox – which is right for you. Tackling asthma, with all its unresolved questions (we still don't fully understand its causes and there is as yet no 'cure'), can seem to be a confusing and at times daunting prospect, but rest assured that there is sensible and easy-to-follow help now widely available, plus telephone helplines and support groups for further advice and information.

So whether you rely solely on orthodox medicine or

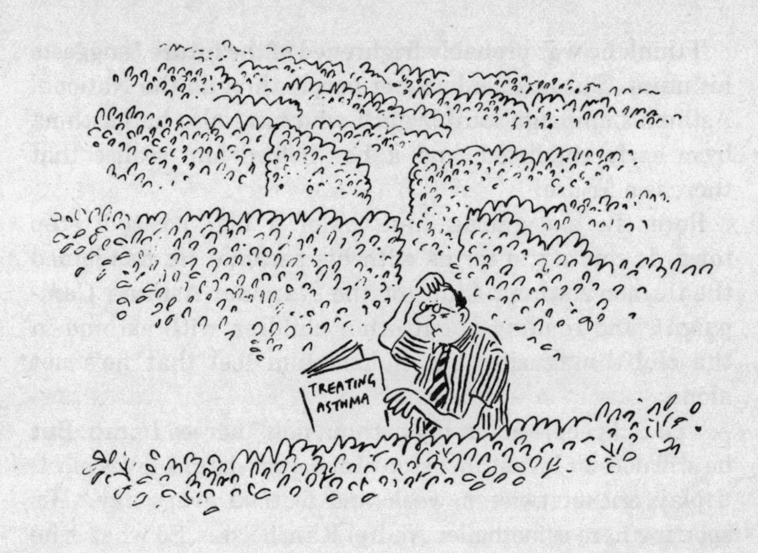

whether you are attracted to the self-help and complementary treatments now available across the UK, there is much you can do – like Janet – to take control of your own health. These days asthma need not put limits on how you live your life.

IMRAN'S STORY

You wouldn't know it to look at him; he is a lively, smiling boy who adores sport. But Imran, now aged eleven, has had asthma since he was a small baby.

'He is still very prone to infections,' says his mum. 'In winter he's on antibiotics regularly.' And until recently, Imran found his asthma hard to accept. 'No one knew about it at school,' he admits. 'If I had to use my inhaler I would do it in private.'

'I think he was probably frightened of the future,' suggests his mum. 'But now he has met people through the National Asthma Campaign local branch who have also had asthma from early childhood, and it has helped him realise that there is a future.'

Recently too, Imran has taken a big, positive step towards coming to terms with his asthma. He has joined the Junior Asthma Club (of the National Asthma Campaign), and reading about other children with asthma in the club's magazine has helped him feel that he's not alone.

'I do tell people about my asthma now,' agrees Imran. But he still doesn't let asthma stop him doing what he loves most: 'I play cricket twice a week and football every day.' His sporting hero is footballer Andrei Kanchelskis. So what is he going to be when he grows up?

'A football player, of course.'

In good company?

In fact, asthma is extremely common. The number of children with asthma in this country has doubled since the 1970s and one in seven schoolchildren now has a diagnosis of asthma. Asthma is now the most common chronic condition to affect children in this country, and in all, three million Britons have asthma.

So what exactly is asthma? There are no simple answers. Asthma is really a condition with a range of causes and effects which we still don't fully understand. But in simple terms, if we have asthma the airways, both large and small, in our lungs tend to become inflamed more easily, usually due to things we breathe in but also to chemicals produced by the body and stressful situations. This inflammation causes a thick, tenacious mucus and narrowing of the airways, which together make it difficult to get air in or out of the lungs.

Our attacks of asthma may be triggered by dust, cats, cigarette smoke, flu, traffic fumes – or simply a gust of cold air. And when this happens, our inflamed airways become narrower as the swelling increases, the muscles tighten and our lungs begin to produce mucus.

'It's like having a heavy weight placed suddenly on my chest,' says Bill, aged twenty-three. 'I start coughing and wheezing and can't finish one breath before I need another. It's often worse at night, in the early morning, or after exercise.'

'I have a really tight chest,' says Tanza, aged ten, 'like I'm being squashed. It's really hard to breathe and I feel tired, breathless and wheezy. It can happen at any time of day but it's worst when I've been running about a lot. It's very annoying.'

But whatever type of asthma you have, it might be of some

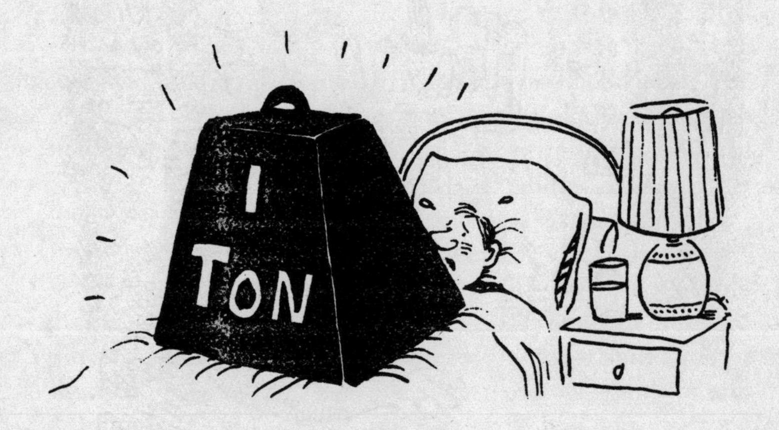

comfort to know that people have suffered symptoms like yours since written records began. And when it comes to treatments, there have been much worse times to have asthma than in the late twentieth century – unless you happen to like powdered live millipedes or tincture of fox's lung, that is!

A SHORT HISTORY OF ASTHMA

Although many of us think of asthma as a very modern problem – perhaps because we connect the rise in asthma with climbing pollution levels – people have been struggling to tackle asthma as far back as civilisation itself. In fact the word 'asthma' comes from ancient Greece where it meant 'panting' or 'gasping'.

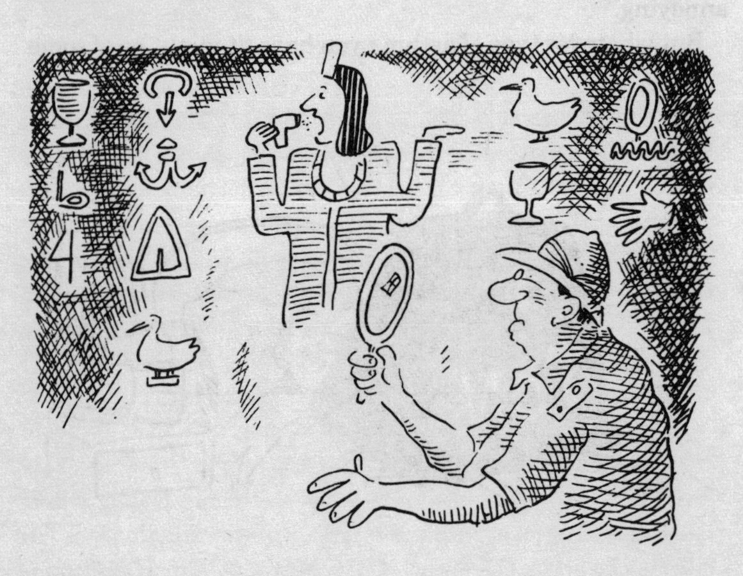

And if you ever feel like chucking away your inhaler or nebulising your nebuliser, spare a thought for the asthma sufferers of long ago who endured 'treatments' – from animal excreta to powdered insects – which would make your toes curl.

According to Ian Gregg of the University of Southampton, (*Southampton Medical Journal*, spring 1991), the Chinese recognised asthma some 4,000 years ago. Their favoured remedy was the Ma Huang plant (a source of the modern drug ephedrine, which has been used in recent times as a treatment for asthma).

The ancient Egyptians also had knowledge of asthma, as a papyrus of 1550 BC makes clear. Their favoured remedy was to inhale an extract of the herb henbane (aka the tobacco plant) which was evaporated on a hot brick. And after Christopher Columbus discovered America in 1492, tobacco again turns up as a prescription for asthma – one angle that today's cigarette companies haven't tried! Even as recently as the early twentieth century, many physicians regarded tobacco as good for people with asthma, and Potter's Asthma Smoking Mixture was a patented remedy which included tobacco.

The ancient Greek Hippocrates – who lived about 400 years before Christ – believed that asthma was caused by 'humours' which flowed from the brain. In someone with a 'phlegmatic' constitution (our modern word 'phlegm' derives from this idea), these humours caused asthma by attacking the lungs. Hippocrates suggested getting rid of the offending humours by various forms of purging – from bleeding to vomiting.

No sex and plenty of chicken soup

His ideas were taken up by the physician Galen whose teachings held sway from 200 AD until the Middle Ages. As late as the sixteenth century, Archbishop John Hamilton of

St Andrews, brother of the Regent of Scotland, was treated for asthma according to Galen's ideas. John Hamilton had consulted doctors from all over Europe. All had agreed his difficulty in breathing stemmed from an overflow of cold and moist humours from his brain. Then Hamilton sent for Girolamo Cardano of Padua, who was reputed to be the best doctor of his time.

But when Cardano came to Edinburgh to observe his new patient he reckoned that it was hot and dry humours – rather than 'phlegm' – which were causing Hamilton's problems. The Archbishop's brain would have to be cooled, decided Cardano, who prescribed regular baths, a strict diet and an irritant ointment to be applied to the skull in order to purge the brain of the evil humours.

And finally, he told the Archbishop to chuck out his feather bed and to sleep on a mattress made of unspun silk. The Archbishop recovered, which suggests that he was allergic to feathers – although Cardano was probably against feathers because he thought they 'heated the brain'.

Moses Maimonides was another physician who was called in to treat the great and the good – in this case, the son of Sultan Saladin of Cairo, where Moses had fled to escape anti-Semitism. His treatments (writes Kay Dempster in *Asthma News*, March 1995, the quarterly magazine of the National Asthma Campaign) included maintaining an even temper, living in a dry climate and avoiding emotional excitement – especially of the sexual variety! And in a remedy which still survives in Jewish mythology today, he prescribed plenty of hot chicken soup.

Stallion dung and dried toad

By the seventeenth century, a number of physicians had begun to question the old Galenic idea that asthma came from humours in the brain – and the first suggestions that 'triggers' such as dust could provoke asthma attacks had started to appear. Jan van Helmont of Brussels (1577–1644) recognised that stirring up dust within the home could cause acute asthma.

He observed of one of his patients: 'As oft as any place is swept all the wind doth otherwise stir up the dust. He presently falls down, being almost choked.'

Sir John Floyer (1649–1734), a physician in Lichfield, observed that asthma could be triggered by a range of factors including changes in the weather, tobacco smoke, metallic vapours, exercise, certain foods – and the sweeping up of dust. Floyer, like van Helmont, reckoned that asthma was caused by 'cramps' or contractions in 'the muscular fibres of the bronchia.'

Meanwhile, remedies for asthma were becoming more and more bizarre. Linctus of fox's lung, stallion dung and dried toad were amongst the cures listed in medical textbooks of the day. One early eighteenth-century textbook recommended a powder made of live millipedes.

It wasn't until quite recently that we really began to get to grips with the causes of asthma. A big step forward came when we discovered that the lungs contained a layer of internal muscle. Physicians realised that when this muscle contracts, it can cause bronchial spasm. The Victorian doctor Henry Salter, of the Charing Cross Hospital, observed that hay, feathers and animals were triggers for asthma, and he recommended strong black coffee as a remedy.

The modern view

The biggest breakthrough of all came in the nineteenth century, when doctors finally put two and two together to develop the concept of allergy. Over the centuries it had been noticed that feathers, dust and flowers could cause strong reactions in asthma sufferers, and then the Victorians noticed that hay fever was connected to the summer months and higher pollen levels. The term 'allergy' was finally coined in 1906.

The nineteenth century also saw the introduction of the first effective drugs for asthma. Out went dried toad and powdered millipede; in came stramonium (derived from an ancient Indian herbal remedy) and atropine (the active principle of deadly nightshade, still used today in the form of ipratropium). Other popular but controversial remedies included opium, arsenic, lobelia, valerian, cannabis, amber and amyl nitrate – many of which were still being used as the twentieth century dawned.

Adrenalin was first used at the turn of the century, and was given by inhaler in 1929. Ephedrine, the active component of Ma Huang, was also prescribed in the 1920s. Caffeine, the active ingredient of coffee (traditionally prescribed for asthma) was found to be a source of aminophylline – available since 1908 as a bronchodilator drug.

In the 1950s the corticosteroid drugs (such as Prednisone) became available. By the 1960s, a derivative of khellin – taken from plants for thousands of years – was developed into sodium chromoglycate (Intal), used by so many asthma sufferers today.

The peak flow meter – which helps many people chart the progress of their condition – was invented at the end of the 1950s. But it wasn't until 1967 that we made a very significant discovery – that the house dust mite (its faecal particles to be more precise) is responsible for triggering so much asthma.

Paradoxically, we have come a long way in terms of

controlling symptoms – but we haven't got very far. Many of the modern asthma drugs are still based on the age-old remedies, while we have yet to find asthma's cause – and asthma's cure.

CHAPTER 2

My Asthma? Your Asthma?

EDWINA CURRIE: A POSITIVE DYNAMO

There aren't many people in this world – public figures or otherwise – who give the impression of being about to burst at the seams with energy and enthusiasm. Edwina Currie, Conservative MP, former Cabinet Minister and candidate in the 1994 European elections – as well as novelist and pundit on issues of the day – is certainly one of them.

When she first arrived at Westminster as an MP she was likened to an eager pupil, hand always up, pencils always sharpened – and a decade later Edwina is still sharp, still eager. It might surprise you then to hear that Edwina has asthma: it might surprise you even more to hear that, in a roundabout way, asthma has been for her a positive spur towards success.

Her condition made itself felt very early on: 'My asthma has always been there,' says Edwina 'although it was not diagnosed as such. I had what was called "catarrh"; in other words I was chesty and wheezy.' But that was no big deal for a child growing up in the big smoke of post-war Liverpool. And apart from missing games at school, it didn't seem to hold her back much; she simply read books instead. As for treatment – 'There wasn't any,' says Edwina simply.

Her 'chestiness' got a little better as she grew into a teenager. A consequence, she thinks, of the Clean Air Act of 1956 which put a stop to the sulphurous smogs of the day. She remembers staying quite well during her school days: 'that could have been because my school had stone floors and no carpets. Nor did we have fitted carpets at home until later in the 1960s,' she says.

I owe my life to modern medicines

It was when she was in her third year at Oxford in 1968 that asthma began to take its toll:

> 'Partly because of the strain of being in a different environment, I became quite poorly, wheezing and coughing a lot and not sleeping properly. In the end I became debilitated, picking up infections easily, and after a particularly bad winter term I was given salbutamol: it was wonderful, it changed everything. I owe my life to salbutamol and my Ventolin inhaler.'

Life took off for Edwina and before long, her career was up and running. But ten years later, after the birth of her second child and a period of generally overdoing it, she came down with a bad case of viral pneumonia. Yet this particular cloud turned out to have a silver lining when her doctor suggested doing a skin test to check for allergies: 'Much to my surprise, it turned out that I am allergic not only to house dust mites, but to . . . feathers!'

Now as luck would have it, Edwina's mother-in-law grew up on a goose farm and bequeathed her quantities of bedding – pillows and eiderdowns – which were literally stuffed with feathers. 'We had a houseful of feathers, which all had to go. They ended up in the guest room, and we started again with new, synthetic pillows and bedcovers which I am very careful to put through the washing machine as often as possible.'

And Edwina has taken the message on board about dust mites too, which thrive on fitted carpets and curtains: 'Our home in Derbyshire is an old stone building and we avoid furnishings which would attract dust mites. My office there has wooden floors and no curtains, while our cottage in France similarly is without fitted carpets.'

Yet it's impossible, for someone with Edwina's lifestyle to avoid the perils of modern interior environments altogether. She has to travel a good deal, and not everywhere she stays is suitable for someone with her type of asthma: 'Hotels drive me crackers! I often ring up in advance and ask for non-allergenic pillows in my room, but that's not so easy when you are going to somewhere like Moscow.'

Even more difficult, however, are private homes:

> 'I once went to stay in an old castle, and I ended up stripping all of the bedding, putting it in the bathroom, and sleeping on the floor. When the maid came in the next morning, her eyebrows shot up. It looked as if I'd completely wrecked the room. But the effect of the bedding on me was awful: I felt all grotty and bunged up for the rest of the next day.'

Asthma clearly hasn't stopped Edwina from pursuing her career, but has it made a difference to what she has done with her life? She says:

> 'Asthma to me is like a light on the dashboard. If I'm overdoing things – too much work, not enough rest and recreation – it shows up as a warning. My chest starts to

> hurt as if my system is saying to me "slow down!". I know that if I ignore that warning I will end up in bed, probably with flu, for at least a week. But if I cancel tomorrow, and instead of working go to a movie or to the gym, I'll be okay.'

Edwina is no couch potato, however, and exercise is a vital plank in her defence strategy against asthma: 'I've been to the gym already this morning, and as long as I use my puffer beforehand, it doesn't bring on asthma.'

I'm fit by most standards

And this former junior health minister is justifiably proud of her fitness:

> 'I am fit by most standards, and my lung capacity is average – which is pretty good for someone with asthma. If I didn't do exercise I would be below par, lacking in stamina. It is essential to keep your lungs clear in a vigorous way. If you are energetic, you stay energetic. The worst thing you can do if you have asthma is slump in an armchair with a cigarette.'

When she's in Derbyshire, weather permitting, Edwina prefers to go for a good three-hour ramble to get herself puffing and blowing, but when she is in London she will go to the gym on average three times a week. 'I like to vary it with swimming and I go jogging in St James's Park too,' she says.

Asthma, she reckons, has only really stopped her in one regard, and that is in team sports: 'It did prevent me doing sport which I regret. Any energetic activity I do has to be on my own so that I can stop and use my puffer when necessary, and then carry on. I am sad to have missed out on that aspect of British culture.'

But what about her job: has asthma been a barrier to achievement?

'No, asthma hasn't stopped me at all. Since that episode of pneumonia which was seventeen years ago, I've been fine. But it did teach me that my asthma is always there. I will still have it when I am an old lady.'

And, she says, there have been two very positive aspects of her asthma which have shaped her life too: 'As a child while everyone else did sports, I sat with my nose in a book. It was thought to be rather eccentric of me, but the end result was that I got a scholarship to Oxford, which I probably would not have got had I been busy playing sports.'

In a curious way, then, asthma has not only helped Edwina to pace herself, but it has helped her to live life to the full: 'You have to develop stamina, both physical and mental, to cope with a chronic disease, and that stamina has also helped me in my job. I now regard asthma as an old, gnarled, warty friend who will tap me on the shoulder from time to time and say – "Hey, don't overdo it!" '

Which – given Edwina's energy level – is probably just as well!

NIAMH CUSACK: A BRILLIANT CAREER

Niamh Cusack has had the sort of career that most of today's young hopefuls can only dream of. Beginning as a professional flautist with the RTE symphony and concert orchestras, she went on to acting in Dublin's prestigious Gate Theatre – and then to starring roles in the Royal Shakespeare Company, followed by some choice parts in film and TV dramas.

Yet in Niamh's childhood anyone might have been forgiven for thinking that – with her breathing difficulties – she wasn't likely to get very far. Niamh reckons it all dates back to a bout of pneumonia which struck when she was a baby: 'I was only six weeks old when I got pneumonia and it left me weaker so that I was susceptible to asthma – which persisted until I was about eleven. It wasn't a hereditary thing, although we do have eczema in our family.'

After the pneumonia, a number of things could set off Niamh's breathing difficulties – such as hay in the countryside, and nervousness: 'I was a nervous child and the asthma came on whenever I got into a state – which I often did when I had music competitions. I can remember the feeling of suffocation, of not being able to find the next breath. It would make me very panicky.'

And Niamh's asthma was, at times, serious enough to leave her unconscious:

> 'A few times it was quite scary to the extent that I occasionally conked out. I remember having to take some horrible-tasting pink medicine, and I also used inhalers. The medicine helped, but I wished there was something which could have stopped the symptoms from coming on.
>
> 'I was off school a lot – I forfeited the official grant to my Gaelic school for three years in a row because I was there so little – and I was always considered to be the weakling in my class.'

That is something that Niamh's friends now think quite extraordinary: 'Anyone who knows me these days sees that I am terribly healthy and strong. I'm the one who goes out with wet hair; who runs four miles a day and who follows a healthy diet.'

So how did Niamh emerge from asthma to her current state of robust good health? In part, she has her mother to thank for that: 'My mother was constantly trying to find a cure for my asthma, and at one stage someone said to her that a wind instrument might help with my breathing. I thought the flute looked like the prettiest instrument to play, so I took it up – and a year later I was free of asthma symptoms.'

Yet there were several different elements in this change for the better, believes Niamh: 'The flute definitely helped my lungs. But it was also my age; I think I was one of those people who have childhood asthma and "grow out of it" at around puberty. It was also partly psychosomatic: I believed the flute would help – and so it did.'

Not only did Niamh's asthma symptoms disappear, but she went on to become a professional flautist: 'I found I had a talent, and from there I've never really looked back.'

I was game to try anything, including acupuncture

These days, Niamh not only has a successful career, but she has a baby son, Calum. And these days too she takes responsibility for her own health by using complementary therapies to keep well. When her asthma went away, she developed eczema, and she has since tried a range of therapies in an attempt to keep that at bay, starting with homeopathy:

> 'Homeopathy is great, but it can be very slow, which can make you feel rather despondent. And I found that it didn't make that much difference to my health. Then a friend said, you must try an acupuncturist and I was game to try anything.'

To begin with she saw the acupuncturist every two weeks, and then every two months – with rapid and dramatic results:

> 'Now, after a year of treatment my eczema has completely disappeared. I do feel that complementary remedies are the way forward for asthma and eczema. Preventive medicine has to be the way through and we should use it before falling into poor health.
>
> 'I had acupuncture while I was pregnant, with a view to keeping Calum as healthy as possible before he came into the world. At only five months he is too little to be treated with acupuncture needles as yet, but I am trying to build up his immune system as best I can. He is a breastfed baby, although he has now started on solids. But if I thought my son was developing asthma it would be hot foot to the acupuncturist. I'm taking Calum to see him next week for preventive care, and for a check up for myself.'

Niamh also takes Chinese herbs which are prescribed by her acupuncturist: 'I boil them up to make an infusion which is quite a rigmarole – and they really taste disgusting! But I only use them when things are bad and they work very quickly.'

Yet Niamh's choice to use complementary medicines doesn't mean that she rejects conventional treatments: 'I still go to my GP as well as using acupuncture and herbs. Conventional medicine is not bad and my GP is very sympathetic to the complementary treatments too. The two have got to work side by side.' As for those other important planks in building good health – diet and exercise – Niamh tries hard to follow a sensible regime:

'I drink decaffeinated tea and coffee as much as possible and I'm quite careful to have a wholefood diet. But although I'm supposed to avoid dairy products I do love cheeses and that aspect does sometimes fall by the wayside.

'I know that asthma can sometimes reappear, but I try to keep myself in the best of health so that I'm as fit as possible to combat any problems – and to make the most of life . . .'

CHAPTER 3

Why Me? Why My Child?

WHAT HAVE I DONE TO DESERVE IT?

'I felt very bitter when I was younger. Why me? Why should I have asthma?' This is how Janet, now in her forties, once felt about her illness.

John Donaldson, author of *Living with Asthma and Hay Fever* and himself a lifelong asthmatic, used to ask the same question:

> 'What had I done to deserve this penalty which at times so diminished the joy of living? The answer may be either simple or exceedingly complicated, depending on how deeply we try to penetrate the mysteries of lung behaviour. It is quite possible to control the illness without bothering at all about the physiology; indeed, the question has no final answer and continues to puzzle scientists who spend their lives trying to supply one.'

For parents too, especially mothers of children with asthma, the question 'why my child?' can be fraught with guilt and self-questioning. Says Marion, mother of fourteen-year-old Laura:

'I've been over and over it in my head: why my daughter – and why *not* her brother? What did I do that might have caused her asthma? I didn't smoke when I was pregnant, but maybe it was mould spores from the old cottage we were renovating when she was a baby? Or maybe it was because I couldn't breastfeed her, or because of dust mites in the dust at home; there was always plenty of that! On the other hand, both my mother and grandfather are asthmatic, although I am not, so perhaps it runs in our family?'

A COMPLEX PUZZLE

Not surprisingly, we are all very keen to know what causes asthma. If we know the causes, not only can we make

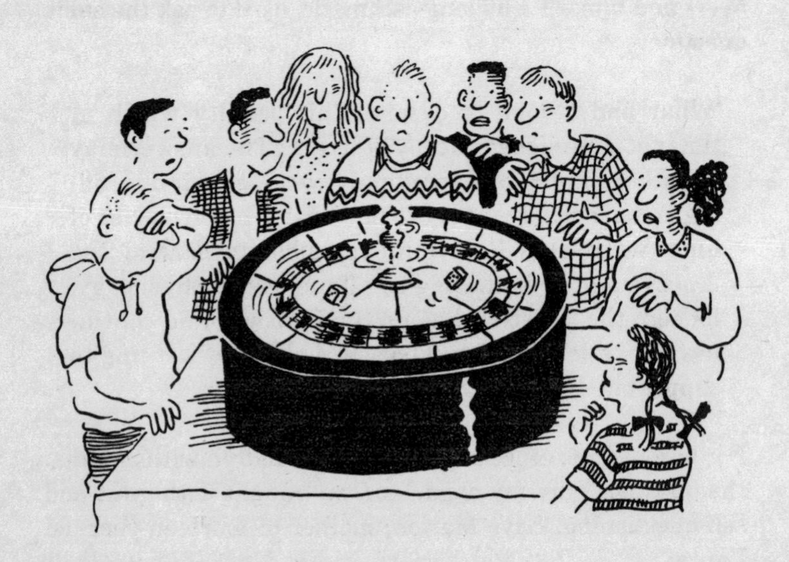

progress towards prevention and 'cure', but perhaps we can shed that tinge of stigma which tends to blame us for our own less than perfect health in this fitness-crazy era. Unfortunately, nothing is simple when it comes to asthma and we cannot yet give a straightforward answer to the questions – why me, why my child? But what we *can* say is that in asthma, there are two major factors to consider. The first is family: all the pointers are that asthma, like the other related allergies, hay fever and eczema, is a tendency which can be inherited.

The second factor is environment: it takes one or more 'triggers' in your home or the outside world to 'switch on' your body's reaction in the form of asthma. Many things have the potential to make your airways narrow – from cold air to cigarette smoke, from chemicals to pollen – and if you have an inherited tendency to asthma, they will narrow with fewer stimuli than the airways of 'normal' people. The major 'triggers' for this kind of reaction, at least as far as children are concerned, are the 'allergens', or substances to which you are abnormally sensitive. Some 80 to 90 per cent of children, and more than half of adults with asthma, are reacting to allergens in their environment.

Chief offenders include the dreaded house dust mite (see page 33); dandruff and saliva from your family pet; pollen from trees, grasses and flowers; mould spores; and some foods (such as milk, yeast and eggs).

Broadly speaking, in very young children the chief cause of asthma seems to be viruses, such as the common cold, rather than allergens. But why asthma is accelerating so fast in the under-fives – faster than in any other age group – is not yet understood, although researchers have their suspicions. One possibility is that it is our terminology which has changed: what doctors once called 'bronchitis' in small children, they now call 'asthma'. Another is that low birth weight and/or the decline in breastfeeding by the previous generation are to blame.

But, apart from occupational asthma (see Chapter 14), there is only one factor which definitely makes it more likely that your child will have asthma and that is smoking. If a mother smokes in pregnancy, or if she or the father smoke when their child is young, then that child is definitely more at risk of developing asthma.

NOW YOU HAVE IT; NOW YOU DON'T

In older children, house dust mites and pets are often the culprits. And once you are into adulthood, allergens again fade out of the picture to be surpassed by infections as a major trigger, together with cold air and a range of chemicals.

In childhood, asthma is more than twice as common in boys as it is in girls – although we don't yet know why. But boys are more likely to lose their asthma in adolescence, so that by the time we reach adulthood the problem is pretty equally shared by the sexes.

Nor does asthma stay constant throughout our lives. Many children who start out with asthma stop having symptoms by the time they reach puberty – which is probably something to do with hormones, although we can't say for sure. By their late twenties, a third of people who once had asthma will have no symptoms, while another quarter will have regular symptoms. The rest of asthma sufferers are somewhere in the middle with usually mild symptoms. But asthma does sometimes return out of the blue and for no apparent reason (although an environmental trigger could be to blame) which is why doctors talk about asthma being 'in remission' rather than being 'cured'.

And increasingly, the experts are suggesting that the first few months of life – and even the months before birth – may be crucial to whether you develop asthma or not. We now know that children who are exposed to high levels of the house dust mite in their first year are more likely than other children to be allergic to dust mites later in life. It could be that if we can avoid contact with these kinds of allergen in babyhood, we can also avoid the allergic reaction to them, which triggers asthma, as we get older.

A SOCIAL PROBLEM?

But not all of us are in a position to avoid the common asthma triggers – and not all of us can follow medical advice which urges us towards a 'healthy lifestyle'. People on low incomes often have less choice than their more affluent neighbours when it comes to important factors such as diet, decent housing, stress, and even the air we breathe.

In a 1994 survey (published in the Archives of Disease in Childhood), researchers found that children in social class E had four times as many asthma attacks as children at the top of the social pile. Smoking, as we have seen, increases the chances of children getting asthma. And smoking, which many people use to cope with stress, is more common in lower income families.

Poor housing is also bad for your health, and if you have the kind of asthma which is made worse by mould spores, a damp home isn't going to do you any good. Exercise is another common 'trigger' for asthma, but what choice do people in high rise blocks have when their lifts are broken except to climb up those stairs?

Simply getting to the doctor can be difficult if you can't afford a car. Not understanding what the doctor – or the literature – means can be a problem for anybody, and especially for families from ethnic minorities. And with the huge hike in the cost of prescriptions in recent years, simply keeping up with your medication may not be all that easy.

Diet, as we all know, is also important to staying healthy so that our bodies are fit enough to fight off infections. But if you are trying to feed a family in bed and breakfast accommodation, without proper cooking facilities, how are you supposed to store, prepare or cook all those nutritious meals?

In this country, the subject of how income affects your asthma hasn't been properly researched but a study which compared the health of East German citizens to that of their wealthier West German neighbours came up with some interesting conclusions. East Germans turned out to have more asthma of the viral kind, probably caused by living in poor and overcrowded conditions. West Germans, on the other hand, had more allergic asthma, which is likely to be because they can afford central heating, double glazing and fitted carpets – in other words, they can afford to turn their homes into havens for the house dust mite which is at the root of so much allergic asthma.

It remains an open question: does a low income make it more likely that you will have asthma – or that your asthma will be more severe? But as we increasingly look to prevention as a way of tackling health problems at their very roots, and as the emphasis in health care moves more and more towards self help, it is a question that cries out to be answered.

A FAMILY AFFAIR?

We have known for a long time that asthma can run in families, but in the 1990s an Oxford-based team of scientists discovered the genetic process which passes allergic asthma and hay fever down from parents to children. These scientists found that a gene on chromosome 11 is the 'blueprint' for making part of the beta chain. The beta chain has been called the 'starter motor for the allergic process' as it begins the process of inflammation when allergens (such as house dust mite particles or grass pollen) come into contact with the cells of your airways.

The Oxford team found three forms of beta chain, but one of them, Leu 181 was found in 17 per cent of the people in the study who had asthma. Leu 181 was always passed on by the mothers in the study. This may explain why women with allergies are more likely than allergic men to have children with allergies.

But despite all this progress there are many questions still unanswered. Why does asthma sometimes skip a generation, so that your daughter or mother may be affected, while you have no symptoms of asthma? Many children have asthma even when no one else in the family has it, although there is likely to be hay fever or eczema somewhere in the family. And what is it that switches asthma on in people who have an inherited tendency – and what can we do to switch it off again?

We don't yet know why it is that more people who have inherited the asthma tendency are now having this condition 'switched on' than in the previous generation. As Dr Martyn Partridge of the National Asthma Campaign puts it (in *Low Allergen Living*, National Asthma Campaign, 1994):

'We know that if a mother smokes during the pregnancy or during the period of early infancy there is an increased risk of her offspring developing asthma. What we do not know is which other factors may similarly increase the risk of a susceptible child developing allergy and asthma. The answer may be in our diet, it may be in the wider environment, or it may be in our homes, and much more research is needed.'

CHAPTER 4

Trigger Happy

WHAT SETS OFF YOUR ASTHMA?

'What brings on my asthma?' ponders Jeffrey, a student, when I ask him this question. 'How long have you got . . .? Just for starters there's the house dust mite; chocolate; dogs; pollen; food additives – I'm allergic to them all. Going from a warm room to a cold one can set it off too.'

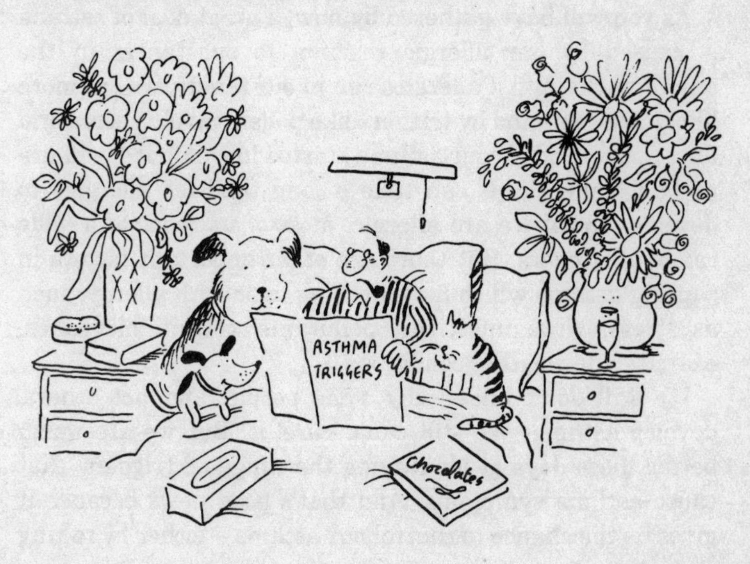

Laura's mother, Marion, finds it just as hard to pin down the 'triggers' of her daughter's asthma (which recently went into remission as Laura reached her teens):

> 'It could have been pollen; it could have been dust mites, or mould spores – we never really knew. But too much excitement certainly set her off. Year after year when she was little Laura missed her own birthday parties – we simply had to cancel them at the last minute because she became so breathless. She missed out on family walks too because cold winds would sometimes cause asthma – but at other times they wouldn't. It was very hard to predict.'

'I don't know why it started in the first place,' says nine-year-old Zoe, 'but when I run about a lot my chest gets very tight.'

As you will have gathered by now, a great deal of asthma is caused by our allergic reaction to substances in the environment, and if allergies run in our family, we are more likely to be affected by triggers like pollen, mould spores and dust mites. And if your asthma started in childhood, you are probably allergic. It can take a long time for allergies to develop, and if we are allergic, most of us react to a wide range of triggers. But there are other important factors in causing asthma which have nothing to do with allergy, such as stress, virus infections, pollutants, certain medicines, exercise and weather conditions.

We still don't know why some people, and not others, develop asthma. We still can't 'cure' it. But we are much better these days at identifying the range of 'triggers' that cause asthma symptoms. And that's good news because it gives us the chance to control our asthma – either by taking avoiding action, or by taking preventive medicine.

This chapter describes the common asthma triggers, starting with the ones which cause you to react allergically, and suggests how you can protect yourself from them. The next chapter looks at the role of medicine in controlling asthma.

BEDFELLOWS FROM HELL

Alas, one of the most important asthma triggers, the house dust mite, is not easy to avoid. This tiny creepy-crawly, invisible to the naked eye, gets virtually everywhere in our modern, centrally heated, wall-to-wall carpeted homes. It doesn't matter how houseproud you are, there are still likely to be a couple of million of them in your bed, not to mention your sofa, your curtains, your duvet . . . and it is dust mite droppings which can cause distressing symptoms in at least three-quarters of people with asthma (for the full, skin-crawling story of the dust mite, turn to Chapter 13).

You could avoid them if you were a time traveller perhaps – as long as you went backwards in time to sleep in a bed of planks in a howling draft. Or if you moved to a monastic cell devoid of furnishings and radiators. But realistically, in today's world there is no getting away from the dust mite altogether, although efficient vacuuming, special bedcovers – and in some cases, chemical mite killers – can keep their numbers down.

With the impossible wisdom of hindsight, the best thing to do is to avoid dust mites when you are a baby, especially between the ages of three months and six months. This is a period in which researchers now believe you first become 'sensitised' to dust mites, laying the groundwork for future allergic response. None of us can put the clock back with our own asthma: what we can do is try to make sure that our children grow up in a relatively dust-mite-free environment. You can't vacuum away the dust mite; it clings on to fabrics with its many little legs. But you can make a significant dent in the amount of dust in your home which – when airborne – will seriously get up a child's nose.

So why not get out that damp cloth, buy a first-class vacuum cleaner – and then get someone else to do the cleaning! When it's finished, throw open the windows for good measure.

BLOWING IN THE WIND

It's tough being allergic to pollen. Especially if you have looked forward all winter to a bit of sunshine and fresh air. Especially if you are the outdoor type who loves nothing better than a ramble in the countryside. But unfortunately, just as our own human sap is rising, so nature sends out billions of the tiny seedlings which get into our airways and which can make summer months a misery.

The pollen season in the UK generally starts sometime in April, reaches its peak in June and July, and dies down by the end of September. It is not flowers that cause most of the trouble as their pollen tends to be carried by insects, but the windborne pollens of trees, grasses and weeds that rise in great clouds during the summer to be distributed across hundreds of miles.

So what can you do to avoid the ill effects of pollen, apart from shutting yourself in the house and missing the glories of summer? Timing your excursions into the garden or countryside can be helpful according to John Donaldson, author of *Living with Asthma and Hay Fever*, who was asthmatic all his life:

> 'In fair weather, pollens rise into the sky during the morning. They descend again in the early evening. So it may be a good plan to open the windows only during the middle of the day. I have doubleglazed the windows of my bedroom as an added precaution, and I close them after 4 p.m. Well fitting outside doors are also advisable.'

The best time to visit your garden, reckoned John Donaldson, is for several hours after a shower of rain has brought pollen down from the sky. And although pollen is released by plants on sunny days, it actually does more damage to your airways in damp weather when it exudes the tiny protein particles which can trigger asthma.

If you are on holiday, or going out for the day, an afternoon at the seaside should be relatively pollen-free because of the onshore breezes – but get home before the wind direction changes in the evening. If you are driving through the countryside, it can help to keep car windows closed too.

Heading for the hills or for northern climes where the season lags behind may also help – as Marion discovered when setting off from the West Country with a wheezing child in the car: 'We weren't sure if we ought to leave home at all because her asthma was so bad, but as we headed up the M5 it started to improve. By the time we got to our holiday cottage in Yorkshire she was fine, and we had a lovely holiday.'

Some other tips from asthma sufferers who react to pollen:

- Increase preventer medication before the pollen season begins.
- Monitor your peak flow levels as the pollen season approaches.
- Avoid areas of long grass.
- Rinse your hair at night during the pollen season.
- To bring an asthma attack under control, try seeking out an air-conditioned office or car.

BREAKING WITH MOULD

Mould spores are tiny pollen-like particles released in their millions by fungi, usually in summer and autumn, and one in twenty people with asthma is allergic to them. Mould grows anywhere warm and damp, from the mulches in your garden to the damp patch on the plaster under your stairs, and it likes to release its spores into damp air, especially at night. As with dust mites, it is nigh impossible to avoid mould spores altogether.

But there are various common-sense measures which can help to keep mould spore levels down in your own home at least. Obviously, tackle any damp areas around the house with appropriate repairs (see also Chapter 13). When decorating, go for paints rather than wallpapers if you are allergic to mould (but not if you react to the chemicals in paint!), and vinyl rather than carpets in damp areas like the bathroom. Clean off mould from windows, tiles and walls.

Air your bedding outside if possible, and again, throw those windows open to get the air circulating around your home. This will help combat damp as well as deterring those dust mites. And don't be a hoarder: that pile of old clothes you keep meaning to take to a jumble sale – but forgetting – could be a haven for mould.

WHAT YOU EAT, YOU ARE?

The whole question of food allergy or food intolerance is still hotly debated in medical and holistic circles. Orthodox doctors say that food allergy is rare as a trigger of asthma, while their complementary colleagues accept the evidence of individuals and get on and deal with it anyway. But whichever way you turn for help, food intolerance is hard to diagnose and you may have to try an 'exclusion diet' – in which you stop eating certain foods while taking peak flow readings (measuring the fitness of your lungs) – to test your response.

There is no doubt that some people, including some people with asthma, do react allergically to certain foods, often with dramatic consequences. We have all heard press reports of people who have collapsed and even died after eating a nut or food that contains nuts. But these are not strictly asthma attacks, although they may involve asthma symptoms.

Allergens in food can be hard to identify (milk for instance, has thirty different proteins of which two – casein and betalactoglobulin – are known allergens). But some are well known, such as the preservative metabisulphite which is found in some alcoholic and some fizzy drinks as well as in some meats and seafoods.

Amongst the long list of foods which may cause an allergic response in asthma are dairy products, alcohol, seafood, yeast and peanuts. Artificial additives in food and drinks, as well as salt, are also under suspicion.

But can avoiding certain foods, or eating certain others,

help you to control your asthma? Again, opinion is divided. If you think you are allergic to a particular type of food, the best thing to do is to avoid it – whether you have medical evidence of allergy or not. However if you, or especially your child, is on an exclusion diet, you are strongly advised to seek help from a dietician to prevent malnutrition.

As for a diet which helps people with asthma, there is some evidence that fish oil supplements can reduce your allergic response. According to *Asthma News* (issue 36), one study has claimed that a diet high in fish leads to less troublesome asthma, which may explain why asthma is rare in Japan.

Whether we have proof of food intolerance or not, common sense tells us that a healthy, wholefood diet, low in food additives, is going to help us maintain good health so that we are in good shape to resist viral infections and to cope with the challenge of asthma.

THE PET THREAT

There are other creatures in our homes which are rather larger and more cuddly than dust mites but which are almost as perilous for asthma sufferers. Cats, dogs, guinea pigs, hamsters, budgies – anything furry or feathered – can be a major source of allergen in your home second in irritant value only to the mite. And heartbreaking as it may be to think of getting rid of Moggy, doctors really do quite strongly recommend it. It might harden your heart to know that 40 per cent of children with asthma are sensitised to cat allergens. And once children are sensitised, even brief exposure to a cat can lead to an attack of asthma severe enough to require medical attention. In the long term too, exposure

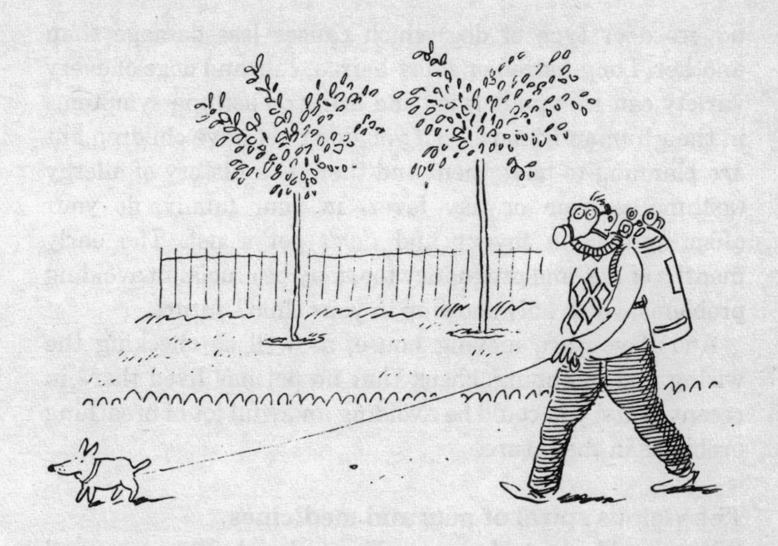

to cats can mean daily symptoms of coughing, wheezing and breathlessness.

The allergen produced by cats is called *Felix domesticus* I, or *Fel d.* I, and it comes from cats' sweat glands. *Fel d.* I sticks to cats' skin and fur, and as it dries out it floats around the air of your home for hours at a stretch. This allergen is particularly persistent and difficult to get rid of. It can even linger in rooms where a cat has been for several years after the animal has gone – which explains why you may start wheezing when you go into a room, even when no cat is present.

Woof woof wheeze

Dogs are a little less hazardous for people with asthma, with only 10 to 15 per cent of children being sensitised to the canine allergen. In dogs, the offending particles are found in dander (dandruff), fur and saliva, and unfortunately there is no breed or type of dog which causes less damage than another. Long-haired or short-haired, cats and dogs of every variety can set up allergies and bring on asthma symptoms in their human friends. So if you don't yet have children but are planning to have them and there is a history of allergy (asthma, eczema or hay fever) in your family, do your offspring-to-be a favour and *don't* get a pet. The early months of life, and pregnancy too, may be crucial in avoiding problems which only show up in your child's future.

And if you are moving house, as well as checking the wiring and plumbing, check that no pet has lived there in recent years: you could be avoiding an awful lot of breathing problems in the future.

The vicious spiral of pets and medicines

What should you do, however, if you already have a pet and someone in the family has developed asthma? As hard as it may sound, the best thing you can do is to give the pet away. If you can't face that, keep it outdoors or let it in no further than the kitchen. It won't thank you, but also try to give it a bath once a week.

If you do manage to give your pet away, instigate a very thorough cleaning regime – preferably with a steam cleaner – to get rid of allergen from all those places where the pet might have been. Experts recommend that you vacuum in places where your pet lived daily for six months, concentrating on carpets and soft furnishings. After that, try not to let other people bring their pets – with attendant allergens – into your home. Even a visit from friends with pet hairs on their clothes can leave allergens on your sofa for a long time to come, and if you have been visiting friends who have pets it makes sense to put your clothes through the washing machine as soon as you get home again.

It all sounds very fussy, and to this pet-loving nation perhaps a bit extreme, but the alternative – a lifetime of asthma and drug treatment for someone in your family – is surely worse. As asthma expert Dr Morrow Brown has put it (*Asthma News* summer 1993):

> 'Find a happy home for the pet, allow the child occasional visits, and everyone will settle into a happier time. The vicious spiral of pets causing allergies which require drugs to mask the symptoms whilst sensitivity increases, leading to yet more suppressive drugs, should never be allowed.'

AND UNCLE TOM COBBLEY AND ALL

There are other substances which can cause an allergic reaction leading to asthma symptoms. Aspirin is known to trigger asthma in up to three in a hundred people, as well as some other pain relievers and medicines such as beta-blockers, non-steroidal anti-inflammatory drugs and some eyedrops for glaucoma. To be on the safe side, always ask your pharmacist whether medicines contain drugs you may be allergic to. And should your doctor write you out a prescription, remind him or her that you have asthma too.

A whole range of chemicals can also cause asthma symptoms (see Chapter 13). Many solvents, glues, paints and treatments used in DIY and home maintenance are irritating to your lungs and over 200 chemical agents used in industry are now known to cause asthma. So if you must use these substances, try to avoid breathing their fumes by working with windows open or work outside if possible.

If you take exercise outdoors, try to avoid those hot summer days when ozone levels are high. An activated carbon filter may help protect you from some polluting gases but not others. And stay away from exhaust and industrial fumes as much as you can.

The non-allergic triggers

As Marion and Jeffrey have testified, there are many and various triggers which can cause asthma in different people at different times and these may change with time as we grow older. Cold air can be a problem for people with asthma, particularly when walking or playing sports on a winter's day.

It may help to put a scarf around your face on cold days which will help warm the air as you breathe in. And make sure you warm up slowly before vigorous exercise, which is good practice anyway in all sports, and use your reliever inhaler. Or avoid the problem altogether by exercising indoors in winter, outdoors in summer.

Air pollution – whether from car exhausts, factory emissions (see Chapter 15) or cigarette smoking – can also cause an angry reaction in your airways. The best advice is not to smoke and to ask others not to smoke near you. It may be hard to ask, but you do have a right to breathe clean air.

Flu, colds and other viral infections can start asthma attacks, especially in small children and particularly in winter. So keep healthy with a good diet and exercise and try to steer clear of people who have colds (which I know is easier said than done, particularly when children are at school!).

Stress can also bring on asthma attacks in some people, so when you feel the pressure building, slow down and perhaps try a relaxation technique such as yoga or Qi Gong (see Chapter 7).

Whatever triggers your coughs or wheezes (and this may change with time and the seasons of the year), identifying the source of the problem enables you to take avoiding action and to take control of your asthma.

CHAPTER 5

Medical Treatments

FINDING YOUR LEVEL

With asthma, there are almost as many levels and forms of treatment as there are wheezy people. Some of us are able to keep our intake of medicines to the bare minimum: others are well aware that modern drugs have literally saved our lives.

Margaret has chronic asthma which developed when she was forty-nine. Her father was a severe asthmatic, and although her daughter Marion has no signs of asthma so far (she does have eczema), her granddaughter Laura has also suffered severe asthma as a child. From this four-generation-long perspective, Margaret is very keen to point out that modern drugs can be life-savers, despite the bad press they are often given:

> 'When I had a really awful attack, panting and sweating like anything, I collapsed on the floor. The doctor came and put me on Prednisolone [a corticosteroid] which probably saved my life.
>
> 'I've now been on Prednisolone for fifteen years (between 5 and 30mgs a day depending on how well I am), as well as inhaled relievers to improve my daily symptoms. I'm sorry to say that I have friends who still really struggle

with their asthma because they are scared of steroids.

'In the past, my father was put on a high dose of the steroid drug cortisone, and when he was taken off it he developed pneumonia. But over the years they've minimised the side effects of steroids.

'And yes, there are side effects when you take steroids in tablet form. I have "thin skin" on my shins. The skin becomes papery and I have to be very careful not to cut myself; some years ago a cut developed into an ulcer. The drug also lowers your resistance to infection and I am slightly prone to minor infections, such as sties in my eyes. I have a flu jab in winter too.

'But I can run up the stairs to my flat on the top floor, and I live a normal life. These days my asthma doesn't limit me in the least.'

Charles, on the other hand, has mild asthma which only bothers him on occasions – such as when he was camping near London last year – and he tries to get by without taking asthma drugs as much as possible:

'I don't know whether it was pollen or pollution, but there was a thunderstorm [which can bring on asthma attacks] and I found myself lying there in my tent, struggling to breathe and feeling frightened. I didn't have my inhaler with me. I only use it about twice a year. I don't like taking drugs for asthma because it seems to me rather brutal, the way they open up your airways. In fact I'm the kind of person who doesn't like to take any medicines unless it's really necessary: I'm concerned about side effects and what drugs do to you in the long term. But on that occasion I wished I did have my inhaler with me!'

However mild or severe your asthma, your doctor will recommend some kind of prescription drugs to help you manage the condition. The aim of modern medicine is to minimise the impact of asthma symptoms on your daily life, and to reduce the risks of lung damage and of life-threatening attacks using the minimum amount of medication. This chapter outlines the kinds of drugs now used in asthma, but it is no substitute for going to your doctor for expert advice tailored to your individual needs.

You may also want to find out what kind of self help is available in terms of holistic or complementary care, in which case turn to Chapter 7.

Much of the information which follows is based on the booklets of the National Asthma Campaign, the national charity which offers education and support to people with asthma and their families, and it describes how asthma is managed using orthodox medicine.

A GREAT RELIEF

There are basically two types of asthma treatments commonly used today. The first type, the 'relievers' or airway openers, relax the muscles around your airways when a 'trigger' hits them and they constrict. Relievers can be taken as a rescue when you feel symptoms coming on or when you expect them to come on, as with exercise. Relievers are usually taken from a blue inhaler and they include the drugs salbutamol (also known by the trade names of Ventolin, Salbulin or Aerolin) and terbutaline (known as Bricanyl). There are also longer-lasting relievers for people with more severe asthma, which can be taken from an inhaler or in tablet form.

The reliever drugs are mostly based on adrenalin, the substance our bodies naturally produce to get ready for action (sometimes called the 'fight or flight' chemical). Adrenalin not only makes our hearts beat faster, it also opens our airways and the modern adrenalin-based drugs are adapted to help the lungs without overstimulating the heart.

Reliever medicines, especially when taken in high doses, can sometimes have unwanted side effects such as shaking hands, nausea and palpitations, but doctors say that although these may be unpleasant, they are not dangerous.

If you need to use your reliever often, or the dose taken does not give you relief for as long as expected, it could be a sign that your asthma is not completely under control so make an appointment to see your doctor.

BETTER THAN CURE?

Useful as relievers can be, they don't treat the inflammation of your airways which is a basic problem with asthma. It is the second type of medicine, the 'preventers', which are designed to do just this.

Preventers, as the name suggests, are taken to stop asthma symptoms from appearing at all. Their job is to combat inflammation so that when you meet a 'trigger', an attack is less likely. They don't give instant results; instead, they have to be used regularly, and you will notice their effects over a period of weeks.

Adults are usually prescribed an inhaled steroid drug such as beclomethasone (known as Becotide or Becloforte); budesonide (known as Pulmicort); fluticasone (known as Flixotide). Sometimes adults take another drug called nedocromil (known as Tilade), and drug companies are working on other preventers which may be available soon.

Children who need preventers are more likely initially to be given a non-steroid preventer called sodium cromoglycate (Intal). This protects against the allergic triggers as well as against exercise-induced asthma, and is the first line of treatment for children with allergic asthma. If sodium chromoglycate doesn't work, however, or if the symptoms warrant, children can also be prescribed one of the inhaled steroids.

A QUESTION OF SAFETY

Many of us are understandably reluctant to take steroids – which are powerful drugs – and many parents in particular are very anxious about side effects and how their children's growth might be effected. It is hard not to associate these drugs with the scare stories we have heard about 'anabolic steroids' which are sometimes used by athletes to improve performance. But the type of steroids used to treat asthma are corticosteroids which are like those made naturally by the body, never anabolic steroids. Doctors will reassure you that corticosteroids are safe in the small doses used in inhaled asthma treatments. There is some risk that your voice will become husky using inhaled steroids, and that you may get a mouth infection called thrush. You can cut down this risk by using a spacer (see page 51), and/or by rinsing out your mouth, spitting out and having a drink or gargle after using the inhaler.

The side effects from steroids are more likely to show up when you take them in tablet form. A course of tablets which lasts only a week or two will have few side effects, according to the National Asthma Campaign, but there are more risks (weight gain, thinning of the bones, raised blood pressure) for people who take steroid tablets for a long time. (Steroids can also be injected by a doctor or a nurse to help someone in an acute asthma attack.)

As Margaret has testified, deciding whether or not to take steroids in the long term (and she has been on them for a decade and a half) is a matter of weighing up the possible risks against the benefits. That is something you need to judge for yourself after taking advice from as wide a range of sources as possible (see Resources section at the end of this book).

THE HARDWARE

These days, asthma drugs tend to be inhaled (rather than swallowed or injected), which means that a smaller amount of medicine can be delivered without delay to your airways. The added bonus here is that – as smaller quantities of medicine are used – the risk of side effects is less too.

Asthma inhalers come in various forms, but the aerosol inhaler or 'puffer' is the most common one for taking reliever and preventer medicines. Asthma medicines can also be inhaled as a dry powder using devices such as the Spinhaler, Diskhaler, Rotahaler or Turbohaler. Or, they can be taken as a solution using a nebuliser machine.

Nebulisers create a mist by blowing air or oxygen through liquid medicine. They are useful for people with severe asthma, and during severe attacks, because they allow bigger doses of medicine to be taken. Tablets can also be given if your asthma seems to be getting out of control and these are usually called Prednisolone or Prednisone. Some relievers, such as salbutamol, are also sometimes given in tablet form.

With aerosol inhalers, you push down the inhaler canister in a 'press and breathe' action to release a dose of medicine. This is forced out as fine particles which you immediately inhale. About half a minute later you can, if necessary, release another dose. It's important, however, to use your inhaler correctly (half of people who use them don't!), and the National Asthma Campaign recommends that you do the following:

- Stand up and tip your head back slightly (to stop too much of the medicine from sticking in the back of your throat).
- Shake the inhaler.
- Breathe out gently, enclose the mouthpiece with your lips and start to inhale slowly.
- Then squeeze the canister quite hard with thumb and forefinger, while you breathe in until you've filled your lungs.
- Count to ten before you breathe out again.
- Ask your pharmacist, practice nurse or doctor to check you are doing it correctly.

Some people keep several inhalers in strategic places around the house or office, so that you don't run the risk of not being able to find one just when you need one.

But not all of us, especially young children, have the coordination needed to 'squeeze and breathe' at the right time when using an inhaler, which is where 'spacers' come in handy. These are plastic containers which you connect to your inhaler so that the medicine is trapped inside the spacer. This offers a 'space' between the inhaler and you to allow time for the propellant chemical to evaporate before the drug gets to you. (Babies and children may need to use a mask together with their inhalers.) Then you can breathe in your medicine as you would normally breathe. The spacer has the added advantage of reducing side effects (such as thrush or a dry throat) from high doses of inhaled steroids. Spacers can be used to give high doses of inhaler reliever to someone having a severe attack. And if you don't have a spacer with you in an emergency, you can make an effective DIY version by making a hole for the inhaler in the bottom of a large disposable coffee cup and placing the open end of the cup over your mouth.

There is now also a breath-activated inhaler. As distinct from the tricky coordination needed to 'press and breathe', this new inhaler has been designed to release its drug once you inhale having clamped your mouth over the outlet.

HELPING YOURSELF

But isn't there a contradiction in terms here: a self-help book giving details of prescription drugs? With many other conditions this might be true: where medicines are concerned, control tends to be firmly in doctors' hands. But with asthma, modern thinking gives control over your medication back to you. Doctors call it 'guided self-management' and really it is a way of empowering patients. The idea is that you are the best person to keep an eye on your own asthma and – within agreed limits – to treat it.

Asthma, as we know, can vary greatly from one day to the next, and rather than waiting for symptoms to develop, you can learn what medicines to take and when. A key part of the process is monitoring yourself with regular checks on the state of your airways. One way to do this is by making a note of your daily symptoms. Some hospitals and GPs will provide you with a diary card to record how you feel and what medication you are taking.

Another, more objective way of finding out if your airways are becoming increasingly narrow or inflamed is to use a peak flow meter. This is a device (not suitable for children under the age of six) which you blow into as hard as you can and the resulting measurement tells you just how much capacity your lungs have at any given time – because how fast you can blow out is directly related to how narrow and inflamed the airways are. If your peak flow readings are going downhill, you will know that your asthma is getting worse and that it's time to take action.

If you have a 'self-management plan' which you have agreed with your doctor, you will be able (for instance) to increase your preventer or take a short course of steroid tablets to tackle your symptoms and bring your peak flow readings back to normal.

But, as ever, do keep in close touch with your doctor or asthma nurse and let him or her know if you begin to take extra medication. Self-management plans, say the health professionals, only work if they are mutually agreed and regularly reviewed.

The National Asthma Campaign publishes a booklet called *Self-Management and Peak Flow Measurement* which includes charts for your doctor or nurse to fill in, plus a credit card-sized asthma management plan for you to keep your own records.

CHAPTER 6

When Asthma Attacks

Asthma attacks can be very frightening, especially to parents of young children: 'I'll never forget it,' says Paul, Becky's dad. 'It was Christmas morning, her first ever, and we rushed her into hospital, not knowing what was happening except that her lips had gone blue. They didn't diagnose asthma until several years later.'

'It was the worst night of my life,' says Marion, Laura's mum. 'She was vomiting at intervals of less than a minute and I wondered if she would survive . . .'

'They are pretty scary,' admits Charles, a twenty-four-year-old computer programmer. 'All you can think about is getting your next breath. It's impossible to go to sleep.'

Asthma attacks can be dangerous, especially when something unexpected happens. Joan, a seventy-one-year-old grandmother, who has had severe asthma since childhood says:

> 'Last winter, I got a chest infection which led to a very bad attack. I always have the phone and the nebuliser by my bed and I woke up fighting for breath. With great difficulty I managed to get up, but the telephone and the nebuliser were on the other side. There was no way I could move from one side of the bed to the other

and so I sat there for three hours. It was really frightening.'

But for most people these days asthma attacks need not catch you unawares. Especially when you can chart the state of your airways from day to day with a peak flow meter, enabling you to predict when an attack is building up. Jeffrey, a twenty-two-year-old student whose asthma started when he was fourteen, says:

'I have two or three small attacks a week. What happens is that my chest will feel tight; I will have pain in my chest and coughing. But I've got a management plan and I'm clear about what I have to do, so I take two puffs of Bricanyl. That normally relieves it.

'If the attack is more serious and I am at around three-quarters of my normal peak flow, a few puffs of Bricanyl doesn't work so I increase my dose. But if my peak flow is down to half of the normal measurement, I start taking oral steroid tablets.

'If my peak flow is still falling after that it's Phone for the Ambulance Time! But that hasn't happened since I've got my management plan. And I've only ever had one attack when someone else has had to phone an ambulance for me.

'It's other people really who feel afraid that I might have an attack: I just get on with life . . .'

TROUBLE ON THE WAY

So how can you tell when an attack is on its way? If you have been taking measurements on a peak flow meter and your

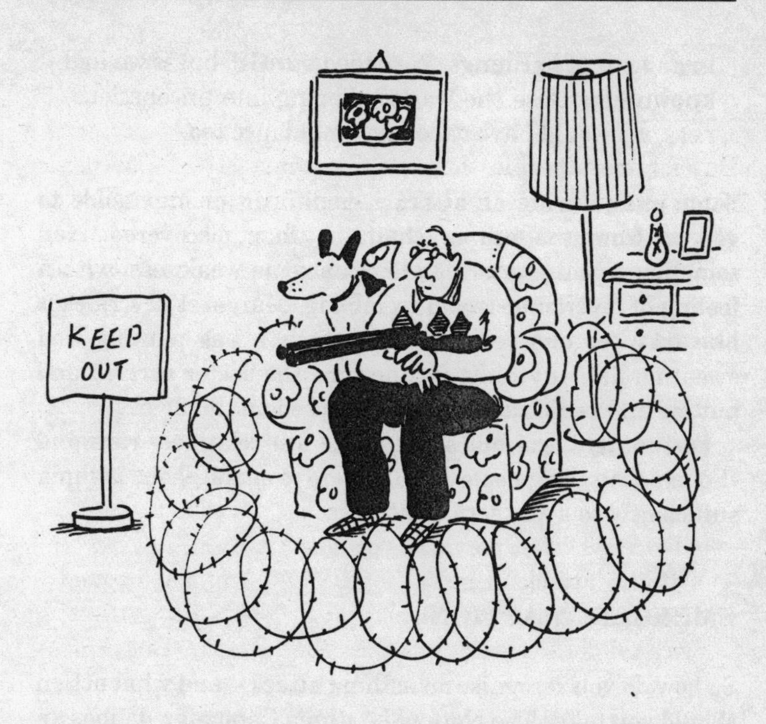

score begins to dip, this is a good indication that trouble is on the way. You may be able to head off an attack by increasing your medication and/or using self-help remedies such as homeopathy or breathing exercises (see Chapter 7).

But when the attack does come, it is often hard to breathe except in short, sharp bursts that you can't control. Sometimes, there is no breath to hear and this condition, called 'silent chest', is a warning of serious danger, as Marion well remembers:

> 'We couldn't hear Laura wheezing so we thought that she was all right – until we saw that she had gone blue. She couldn't even speak because so little air was going

in and out of her lungs. We called our GP, but if we had known how close she was to slipping into unconsciousness, we would have called an ambulance too.'

Sometimes, during an attack it is difficult or impossible to get up from the bed or chair, as Joan discovered. And sometimes, you are in a state of extreme weakness, with a feeling of feverishness and trembling. Margaret describes it like this: 'In one really awful attack I was panting and sweating like anything. By the time the doctor arrived and put me on Prednisolone, I had collapsed on the floor.'

Fortunately, examples like these are relatively rare and the majority of people are able to control their asthma sufficiently to avoid serious attacks.

EMERGENCY ACTION

So how do you recognise an asthma attack – and what action should you take? The National Asthma Campaign defines an asthma attack as when the reliever treatment is not rescuing you from breathing difficulties after the first 5–10 minutes of taking it. In their booklet *Take Control of Asthma*, they suggest you take the following steps:

- Take a reliever again after 5–10 minutes.
- Try to stay calm: relax as much as your breathing will let you.
- Sit in a position that you find comfortable, do not lie down.
- Rest your hands on your knees to help support your back.
- Try to slow your breathing down as this will make you less exhausted.
- If the reliever is still not working, call for help.

The question of when to ask for help – and from whom – is always a vexed one for people with asthma and their carers. As Nicola's mother Sylvia puts it: 'She'll be sitting bolt upright all night in an asthma attack, and for me the worry is, is she bad enough to take in to hospital? Shall I call the ambulance or call the GP?'

But asthma is so variable that there is no 'right' or 'wrong' answer here; almost every situation needs to be judged individually. It can help, however, to discuss this question with your GP as a part of your self-management plan. At a certain stage of an attack (as agreed with your doctor) you will either need to call your GP, or make your way to casualty, or call an ambulance.

If you live in the country for instance, it can be quicker to call a local doctor than to call the ambulance. But if you are having difficulties getting through to your GP – or you are not at home when an attack strikes – don't hesitate to call an ambulance.

John Donaldson, who had asthma all his life, wrote in *Living with Asthma and Hay Fever* that – even in a severe attack – carers need to be aware that the person with asthma may be feeling reluctant to 'cause a fuss': 'When onlookers suggest sending for the doctor, we are likely to shake our heads while secretly hoping that this has already been arranged.'

His practical suggestions about how other people can help include providing a pencil and paper so that the person with asthma can write down what they might need – a drink of water for instance, or a trip to the loo. In addition:

> 'all medicines should be at hand, to enable us to make a selection . . . We want help to be near, but not be alarmist or insistent. When the ambulance arrives, it

> may help to take a dose of nebulised salbutamol (or terbutaline) before being asked to make the difficult journey down the stairs and along the path in the cold, polluted air.'

And with time and experience, people who have asthma can gradually get on top of the situation, knowing exactly what to do if and when asthma attacks: 'I learned by trial and error how to cope,' says Joan, the veteran of seven decades of asthma. 'I now know how to look after myself. I keep a constant watch on my symptoms using a peak flow meter – and I can face a lot of things which I couldn't face before.'

CHAPTER 7

Self Help Through Complementary Treatments

A WIDER VIEW OF HEALTH

Most of us are very thankful to have the choice of taking modern asthma medicines. The bad old days when doctors didn't want us to become 'dependent' on asthma drugs have more or less gone, and these days we are more likely to be encouraged into 'self-management', watching our own symptoms and deciding on our own level of medication.

But modern medicine as we know it didn't emerge with a thunderclap, new and fully formed, some time earlier this century. Many of the asthma drugs which we take today have been known about in their original plant form for thousands of years (see Chapter 1). And we are becoming increasingly aware that western allopathic medicine – which treats symptoms of illness once they have appeared rather than preventing disease or tackling its causes – does not have all the answers.

More and more these days we are interested in using different types of remedies – the complementary or holistic treatments – as well as the orthodox asthma drugs. And while many of these remedies have not been scientifically tested in the same way as modern drugs (the huge profits to be made from prescribed drugs have something to do with

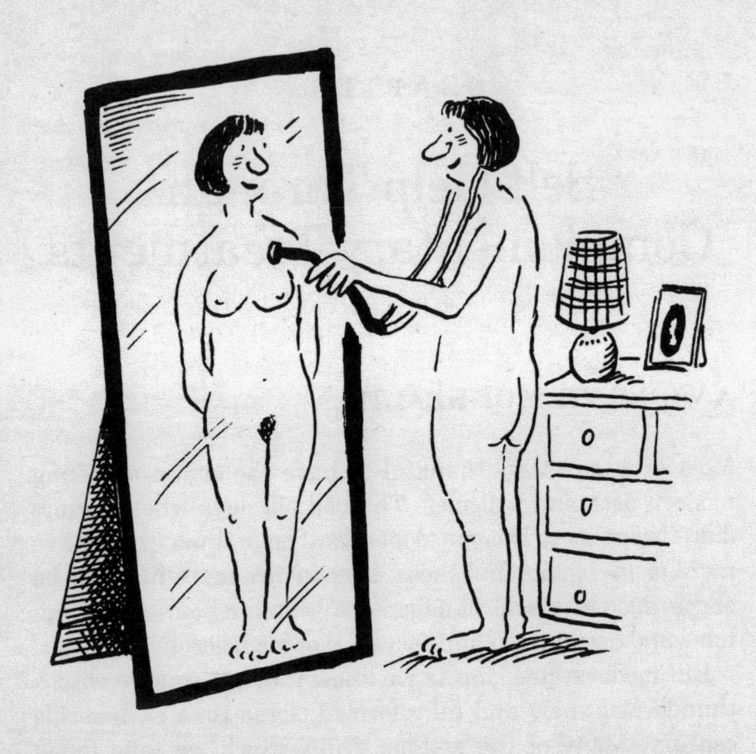

that!), some of them – like acupuncture – have been tried and tested by generation after generation of people over thousands of years.

What's more, many of the complementary therapies try to address the cause of a health problem and how it is a part of the whole person, rather than simply treating (some would say suppressing) symptoms. Many are also cheap, safe and easy to use and without the unpleasant, sometimes dangerous, side effects of some modern drugs.

Other holistic therapies, such as yoga, are clearly 'self-help' therapies in which we take responsibility for our own health. And there is evidence that when people use complementary therapies, they can often cut down on their intake of orthodox asthma drugs.

There is something else about certain complementary treatments which scientific testing doesn't usually measure: they can be positively enjoyable in themselves. After all, how would you rather spend the morning: in a modern hospital ward/doctor's surgery or lying on a couch being massaged with deliciously scented oils? I reckon the aromatherapy wins hands down (as it were) although I'd still want the option of modern drugs in case of an asthma attack.

This chapter, then, is about some of the complementary remedies that people in this country today are turning to as a part of their quest for control of their own asthma.

Richard: going deeper into asthma

Richard, a radio broadcaster now in his mid-thirties, first developed asthma as a teenager. After a few years, however, his condition went into remission, and it wasn't until a bad chest infection laid him low a few years ago that his asthma showed up again:

> 'No one else in my family has asthma, so it came as quite a shock the first time around. But then fortunately it went away – until quite recently. Now I find that exercise, stress, or winter colds will set it off again. My doctor prescribed a Ventolin inhaler and I have a few puffs of that from time to time. But I prefer to use various holistic therapies, and together with the prescribed drugs, these are keeping my symptoms well under control.'

Richard attends the 101 and Good Health Clinics, leading holistic treatment centres and with their main clinic in

London. Treatment has to be paid for: consultations cost from £30 upwards, but the clinic has a long-standing reputation and is used by Tina Turner, George Harrison and the occasional member of the Royal family amongst others! I talked to the 101 and Good Health Clinic's Medical Director, Dr Rajendra Sharma, about holistic treatments for asthma and about Richard's condition in particular. According to Dr Sharma:

> 'The orthodox medical view is that Richard had an infection when he was younger which triggered a prolonged inflammatory response in his lungs. This response is now triggered when he takes exercise, experiences stress or catches cold. Of course there is truth in this view, but orthodox medicine stops there, whereas we go further and ask – why is it that this particular person's body has made his lungs oversensitive?
>
> 'When we take the holistic view of mind, body and soul as interconnected, we see that asthma happens when there has been some form of psychological or emotional repression which sets up blockages in the body. In Richard's case, an alcoholic mother and violent father caused a lot of powerful feelings which Richard, as a child, learned to keep hidden.
>
> 'He wanted to scream and shout because he knew that behaviour within his family was not as it should be. But as a child he couldn't express that; he had to repress it. Imagine what that feels like: his lungs pulled in air, but he didn't know what to say . . . so his breathing halted.'

And that, argues Dr Sharma, is rather like what happens in asthma: 'The holistic view is that his mind saw problems; his body reacted and his soul now keeps the problem going into the present. If we were simply to treat the body, we would not be able to cure Richard.'

'Cure?' I ask Dr Sharma, surprised to hear that magic word. 'Cure is not a term which orthodox medicine uses when it comes to asthma: the received wisdom is that there is no cure . . .'

He smiles:

> 'Of course they say that. Nobody has found a drug to cure asthma because the drug companies would lose far too much money if a "cure" were found. Think how much revenue they get – hundreds of millions in this country alone – from the quantities of drugs prescribed to people with asthma. A "cure" would put an end to that.'

HOMEOPATHIC HELP

But is there a 'cure' available through holistic treatments, I ask? Certainly, there is no single remedy which puts an end to asthma once and for all, and conventional doctors argue that clinical trials – with a few exceptions – have been inconclusive when it comes to asthma. Homeopathy, however, is a form of treatment which is now well documented as helping to reduce asthma symptoms and enabling people to cut down on conventional drugs, and a recent trial at Glasgow's Homeopathic Hospital has confirmed much of the positive evidence.

The long-term aim of homeopathy is not just to control symptoms; it is to restore health so that you can eventually do without drugs or remedies. This can be a slow process and to get there, you need to see a professional homeopath who will tailor your treatment to your unique needs. (It can be especially successful with children who are more than happy to take the little sugar pills, and who often respond with remarkable speed!)

Homeopathy is a system of medicine in which 'like cures like', and minute amounts of homeopathic remedies are given to stimulate the immune system to fight illness in much the same way that vaccinations are given in orthodox medicine. The difference is that homeopathic remedies are without the toxic side effects of many modern drugs. Homeopathy has long been popular with the Royal family – which may or may not encourage you to give it a try!

Unlike prescriptions for conventional medicine, however, it's not possible to say exactly which asthma remedy will suit you. In homeopathy, the practitioner asks, which remedy suits the individual? Depending on many factors, including your personality type and the type of asthma, you could be given any one of about eighty remedies.

TREATING THE WHOLE PERSON

To give an idea of how a holistic practitioner would tackle an individual case, I asked Dr Sharma how he had treated Richard, and with what results? To start with, Dr Sharma (who is a qualified homeopath as well as a GP) advised Richard to keep taking his orthodox medicine (Ventolin) as prescribed while he looked for the cause of the asthma and found ways to help him cut down on his drug intake:

> 'Richard, as a result of the emotional strains of his childhood, had developed a blockage in the energy

flow through the mid-line of his body. I prescribed a homeopathic remedy called Calcarea Carb to deal with his physical symptoms of constricted airways and too much mucus, as well as to help release his repressed emotions.

'But asthma is a potentially lethal condition and we insist that our patients must be under the care of an orthodox doctor – either myself or their own GP. I stress that homeopathy is not a substitute for orthodox medicine, and it is also important to have a consultation with a qualified homeopath rather than to self-prescribe.'

As we have heard, there are many homeopathic remedies which can be used for asthma, but the ones which Dr Sharma commonly prescribes include Aconite (when asthma is sudden or violent, with a restless, dry cough); Ipecac (for sudden onset asthma with anxiety and a feeling of weight on the chest); Thuja (for asthma attacks in children, or when asthma comes on in the afternoon, in the cold or the damp). And at the start of an asthma attack he says, a useful emergency remedy is Aconite 6X (four pills every fifteen minutes) while you await your doctor's assessment.

At the 101 Clinic, people with asthma, including Richard, are always offered some sort of counselling to explore the emotional and psychological roots of their asthma. Children benefit especially from art therapy which helps them express difficult feelings in a non-verbal way.

Breathing exercises – either yoga, or the Chinese system of exercise and breathing called Qi Gong – are also offered at the 101 for people with asthma. Dr Sharma believes these can benefit everyone, a view borne out by scientific research.

Richard has certainly found that they help him: 'I practise yoga breathing exercises whenever I feel asthma symptoms coming on and I find them very effective. I am sure they have helped me to keep my use of Ventolin to a low level.'

Breath control

Yoga is a venerable Eastern form of health care used to establish harmony in mind, body and spirit which dates back some 3,000 years. Apart from promoting relaxation and suppleness, one of its key elements is to use control of the breath to achieve fitness and good health. And as asthma is essentially all about breathing, yoga has much to teach us.

In the West we are more inclined to think of yoga as a form of exercise than as a kind of medicine, and so you are more likely to find a yoga teacher at a local night class than at a health clinic, and there is no register of qualified practitioners.

In yoga you learn 'postures' or positions, in which your body is stretched as far as you find comfortable – which makes it suitable for all age groups. The breathing exercises not only induce deep relaxation which combats stress, but they help to strengthen your immune system and increase your energy.

There is good evidence that yoga helps people with asthma. One study published in the *British Medical Journal* reports that asthmatics who practised yoga had fewer symptoms and needed fewer drugs than a group who stuck to conventional medicine alone.

Treatment that wins on points

Another ancient form of health care, practised in China for many thousands of years, is acupuncture. It sounds and looks rather alarming to untutored Western eyes: long thin needles are inserted into your body at strategic points along the meridians (pathways) along which your 'chi' (vital energy) is said to flow.

Although it can be rather unnerving to watch a needle disappear into your body to the depth of several inches, a skilled acupuncturist (and it is essential to go to a well-qualified professional; see Resources section) will do this without hurting you. As with most complementary therapies, we have little 'scientific' proof of how acupuncture works: yet the Chinese have been practising acupuncture successfully for thousands of years and on millions of people.

For asthma, the acupuncturist will work on adjusting the chi through the lung, bladder, colon or heart meridian. The long-term aim is to control the asthma without using medicines. Asthma attacks are treated by inserting a needle at the 'Ding Chuan' point, just below the neck, amongst others.

Working on the same principles as acupuncture, 'acupressure' is a therapy which works by rubbing or pressing key points along the meridians rather than by inserting needles. As such, you can sometimes have a go at it yourself. Dr Sharma suggests you can practise self-help for asthma by applying pressure to one of the various points on your body known as 'lung points'. One of these is in the mid-line of the body, two fingers-widths upwards from the bottom of the sternum (the breast bone). Another is below the knee: 'With the knee bent,' says Dr Sharma, 'find the prominent part of the large bone (the tibia) below the knee; move to the side and outwards; find the gap between that bone and the smaller bone (the fibula) and massage, pushing downwards.'

Another acupressure point which can be pressed by a friend or family member is on either side of the spine, one finger-width down from the top of the shoulder blade. Again, press inwards and downwards.

Sensitive to food?

There are other therapies available through clinics like the 101 which can help individuals with asthma. Some people find that hypnotherapy can help them to feel more calm and relaxed so that asthma attacks, when they do come, are less serious.

Reflexology, the deep massage of the feet which helps to relieve symptoms in corresponding parts of the body, may also give relief from symptoms of asthma – as well as making you feel wonderfully relaxed!

But if someone is not responding to these treatments, says Dr Sharma, then it is time to look for food allergies or, as he prefers to call it, food intolerance:

> 'The orthodox view is that there is no evidence that foods can cause asthma. However, there have been trials using exclusion diets (cutting out certain foods) which show that one in ten children are sensitive to certain foods – and excluding these foods from their diet will help their asthma.
>
> 'Wheat, milk and refined sugar can cause the release of histamines (the chemicals involved in allergic reactions). We suggest excluding the following foods from your diet for six weeks to see if your symptoms improve: cow's milk; sugar; caffeine; alcohol; oranges; apple and orange juice from cartons. We also use a Vega or Bioresonance machine, to test for food intolerance.'

Proof of the pudding

So how has Richard fared in his quest for a holistic solution to his asthma? He says:

> 'The mainstay of my treatment has been homeopathy, combined with Qi Gong breathing exercises. I've had

counselling too to unearth some long-buried feelings. If I get a bad cold I go back to the 101 for a course of acupuncture and some Chinese herbal medicine, which does the trick.

'It's a long and continuing process, but I like the sense that I am really getting to the root of my asthma, rather than simply dealing with the symptoms. It is reassuring too that the remedies I have used at the 101 Clinic don't have toxic side effects.

'These days I feel my asthma is well under control. I only use my Ventolin inhaler when I exercise hard, and I've been healthy and in good spirits for some time.'

CHAPTER 8

Making Babies, Having Babies

MAKING WHOOPEE?

It's a special night out for you and your beloved. Dinner perhaps, with flowers and candles. And when you get home it's all soft lights and sweet music. Time to head for the bedroom . . . Thus far a familiar scenario. But in the bedroom things are getting rather steamy when – cough, cough, wheeze, oh no! – asthma has raised its ugly head.

Alas for some people, exertion in bed – like exertion anywhere else – can bring on an asthma attack. But there's

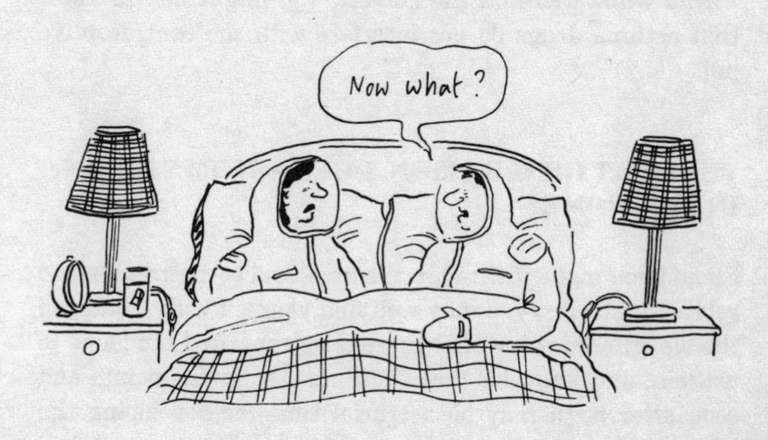

no reason why this should spell death to romance: a puff of reliever medicine (such as Ventolin) before you get carried away will help to keep your airways open.

Another bed problem may be that bouncing on your mattress causes a cloud of dust mite allergens to rise up around you and when there are up to 2 million dust mites keeping you company, that can be a serious drawback to sex. Again, a dose of reliever medicines should see you through.

And spare a thought for those who may be worse off than you in the bedroom department. It is a rare condition, but some women are allergic to their partner's sperm, which means that after having sex they will develop a general allergic reaction including asthma. The symptoms may be immediate, or they may take days to show up, which makes it hard to get to the root of the problem. But the simple expedient of using a condom can help identify, and avoid the allergic response (although a special non-allergenic condom may be necessary). In the long term, however, women with this problem may need to see a specialist.

And while we're on the subject, you might like to know that asthma drugs do not interfere with the contraceptive pill.

THE NEXT GENERATION: DOES ASTHMA BEGIN IN THE WOMB?

Should you make it through the minefield of mattresses and related problems, you may well find yourself with a baby on the way. So knowing that there is an inherited tendency to asthma, and knowing that those months in the womb and soon after birth may be a crucial time for developing the asthma tendency, what can you do to help your unborn grow up as healthy as possible?

For women, the one sure thing you can do to protect your child from asthma is – don't smoke. Maternal smoking is one of only two proven causes of asthma (the other being exposure to occupational hazards, see Chapter 14). Low birth weight, stopping breastfeeding early and family size are other family factors which have been looked at as possible causes of asthma, but none of these has turned out to be as important as smoking.

The allergy to house dust mites may also develop in the unborn child during pregnancy or in the first months of life. This response may lie hidden for many years before the symptoms of asthma develop, but how can you avoid your baby becoming sensitised in the first place?

Dr Jill Warner, the National Asthma Campaign's Senior Research Fellow at Southampton University, writing in *Low Allergen Living* magazine, makes this semi-serious suggestion:

> 'The ideal solution would be to send all pregnant women to environments where house dust mites do not exist – such as the special schools for allergic asthmatic children which are at high altitudes – during their pregnancies and the babies' first year of life, in the hope of preventing the development of allergic disease.
>
> 'As this is impossible for most of us, we need to consider whether we can treat our own homes in a way which will recreate the environment found in such institutions.'

In other words, we need to aim for a low-allergen living environment (see Chapter 16), which means chucking out the carpet and curtains for lino and blinds, using dust mite-proof barriers on our bedding, opening the house to plenty of fresh air and finding a nice new home elsewhere for Moggy or Rover.

There may be a range of factors influencing the tendency to asthma in the womb and in babies – from dust mites to diet, from our home environment to the gases from gas cookers. Apart from smoking, we don't yet know for sure. But the safest course is to build up our own (and our baby's) health by eating plenty of fresh vegetables, by reducing our intake of processed food, and by including fish (especially oily fish) in our diet at least twice a week.

The good news is that *your* asthma should have no ill effects on the health of your unborn baby, unless you are unfortunate enough to suffer such a severe asthma attack that you experience a dangerous shortage of oxygen. This can sometimes lead to the baby having a low birth weight, and – very rarely – to the tragedy of stillbirth.

And it could be that your second, third, fourth (fifth? sixth?) child has some special protection which your firstborn lacks. According to *Asthma News*, researchers in Germany have found that in large families, firstborns are more likely to develop allergies. Some 7,600 nine to eleven year-olds were tested for allergies and those with the most siblings had less allergy. Researchers are speculating that today's small families could be a factor in the rise of allergies in children.

THE DILEMMA OF DRUGS

Since the Thalidomide tragedy of a generation ago, we have all – doctors, drug companies and parents alike – become extremely cautious about taking any kind of drug during pregnancy, especially the early months of pregnancy when the foetus is particularly sensitive to harm. Naturally enough, this leaves women who have asthma on the horns of a dilemma. What do you do – as someone who takes reliever and preventer drugs regularly – if you are pregnant or planning to become pregnant? Mary, mother of a three-year-old daughter and a baby boy says:

> 'They say it's okay to take these drugs. And for the most part I am happy with the drugs that I take for asthma – I'm on Bricanyl and Pulmicort – but I do have lingering worries about them, who doesn't? They say they are safe now, but in twenty years' time they may withdraw them.
>
> 'Yet I have no evidence that they are not safe, and really, I've got no choice. I can't afford to get alternative treatment. And the modern world is full of hazards that our children have to live with from the fumes in the air to pesticides on our food. So I carried on taking my asthma drugs – as my doctor recommended – while I was pregnant and, touch wood, my daughter is as fit as a flea so far. As for my son, he was 8lbs 14oz when he was born; a whopper!'

Dr Martyn Partridge, Chief Medical Adviser to the National Asthma Campaign, has seen many women who stop taking their asthma drugs when pregnant because of worries about harming their baby. But he argues that the dangers of uncontrolled asthma to the baby are far greater than any danger from asthma drugs:

> 'No one can be 110 per cent certain about the safety of drugs, but in the doses we give there are no significant

side effects. The biggest danger to mother and baby alike is from poorly controlled asthma. There is nothing worse than a bad attack at the beginning of a pregnancy caused by mothers unnecessarily stopping their inhaled treatments. The usual asthma drugs, including the steroids, are safe and should be continued in pregnancy.'

HOW DOES ASTHMA AFFECT YOU IN PREGNANCY?

'I felt that my asthma was better when I was pregnant,' says Mary, 'but I was worried about going into labour. My God! What if the stress and strain of giving birth sent me into an asthma attack? But although I had a twenty-hour labour – I had gas and air and a Pethidine injection – I didn't have any asthma symptoms at all.'

But Mary need not have worried about asthma in labour, according to Dr Martyn Partridge: 'Of course the whole thing may be a bit tense, but generally speaking there is nothing to worry about here. I know of no evidence that labour brings on asthma symptoms, and there is no reason why women with asthma can't have epidurals or any of the usual pain relief.'

As for pregnancy improving asthma symptoms, some women seem to feel better, others worse, and some remain much the same. 'There is no evidence one way or the other,' says Dr Partridge. It is true, however, that some women find their asthma is worse before a period: 'If your asthma seems worse premenstrually,' suggests Dr Partridge, 'you can check this by using a peak flow meter. If it is worse, you may benefit either by increasing your usual medication, or by taking progesterone hormone therapy.'

Beware of taking medicines for period pains which contain aspirin or other anti-inflammatory type painkillers, however; these could make your asthma worse. If in doubt, ask the chemist.

ASTHMA AND NEW MOTHERS

Unfortunately for Mary, now the mother of a three year old and a newborn, her asthma has not been improved by the stresses of life as a new mum:

> 'It's definitely got worse since the children were born. The more tired I am, the more wheezy I am. And as my first child rarely slept, I was in hospital with asthma about once a month when she was little.
>
> 'Before the children were born I was on Becotide 50 and a Ventolin inhaler. But after they were born I was put on Becotide 100. I was also given half a dozen week-long courses of Prednisolone in the first year of my daughter's life. That was a worry because I was breastfeeding and who knows what might be going into my breastmilk, but they told me not to worry.'

Again, Dr Martyn Partridge is reassuring: 'The only drugs we are a little bit concerned about when it comes to breastfeeding are the theophyllines which can make children irritable – and continuous, high doses of Prednisolone.' But generally speaking, doctors advise that there is no reason to stop taking inhaled asthma drugs while you are breastfeeding, because such small amounts are absorbed by your body that only negligible amounts will appear in your breastmilk. Using a spacer will reduce the amounts even more.

And there is no doubt that breast is best for your baby in all sorts of ways. Scientific studies have not proved that breastfeeding protects against asthma in particular, but they have proved that it protects against asthma when it runs in families.

'It is better for babies to be breast fed if possible, particularly where one or both parents are atopic or have asthma,' according to Dr Mark Levy *et al.* in their book *Asthma at Your Fingertips*. 'Breastfeeding needs to continue for around six months to reduce the chances of the baby becoming allergic to cow's milk and then developing eczema.'

Breastfeeding also helps to improve a young child's resistance to viruses such as the common cold, which are the most common trigger for asthma in children, particularly in those under one year of age. So the old slogan 'Breast is Best' still holds true – and all the more when it comes to tackling asthma.

CHAPTER 9

Asthma And Your School-Aged Child

For Tanza, it began at the age of nine after a series of winter colds. 'One morning she woke up and she was struggling for breath,' says her mum, Sally. 'I took her to the doctor, and when he got her to blow into the peak flow meter, her reading was only a third of what it should have been.'

Tanza and her mum went home with prescriptions for preventer and reliever medicine – and with the knowledge on Sally's part that there had been a significant change in their lives. 'It's painful, as a mother,' says Sally 'to hear your child diagnosed with something which could affect her for the rest of her life.'

It is the long-term nature of asthma and the prospect of taking drugs every day – perhaps forever – which can be so difficult for parents to accept. But for Tanza, so far, life goes on much as before – except that she has to try to remember to take her medicines. Today's children see asthma as no big deal. Says Tanza: 'There are three other children in my class who have asthma, and some of them have it really badly, much worse than me.'

ARE WE THE ASTHMA GENERATION?

Tanza is quite right in spotting that asthma is now a common problem: an estimated one in seven schoolchildren, one million in all, now have asthma in the UK. (Whether their asthma is more severe than it used to be is still a matter of debate.) On top of that number, another half a million under-fives also have 'asthma-type' symptoms – although doctors disagree on what should be called 'asthma' and what is just 'wheeziness' or 'bronchitis'.

Asthma causes more days off school than any other condition. More children are admitted to hospital with asthma than with any other condition, and, tragically, every ten days a child dies of asthma in this country.

When asthma does show up in children it can be mild or serious. Some will have symptoms every day: others will go for long periods without any symptoms until a 'trigger' such as a virus or a furry animal sets the asthma off.

Many children suffer from sleeping difficulties and tiredness which can make them tetchy and interfere with their concentration during the day. (Where parents have lost sleep through being up in the night with a coughing child they can get pretty tetchy too!) And unfortunately, many children will also suffer asthma attacks which call for emergency medical help.

The symptoms of asthma in children certainly look the same as in adults: children will often cough and/or wheeze, especially at night or after exercise. Your doctor will probably prescribe an inhaler to relieve the symptoms and your child may also need to take preventer medicines daily. But asthma in children, especially young children, may not be simply a junior version of what afflicts their mums and dads. New scientific studies in the UK show that asthma may not be a single disease, but that there are at least two types of childhood asthma. According to the National Asthma Campaign report on childhood asthma *The Asthma Generation*, these two types have different causes and different effects.

In very young children (see Chapter 10), asthma attacks are usually caused by colds or other virus infections and they have nothing to do with allergic reactions. This kind of asthma tends to disappear as children grow up.

The second kind of asthma is the allergic kind and it runs in families where there is a history of asthma, eczema or hay fever. People with this kind of asthma have a genetic tendency to allergy, which is then set off by exposure to allergens such as house dust mite droppings. 'Sensitisation' to allergens is thought to take place in the early months of babyhood, or even before birth – although it may be years before its effects show up as asthma.

The whole family is affected . . .

Nicola's asthma certainly runs in the family – her younger sister is also asthmatic – and she has also had eczema. 'The asthma was part of a severe allergic reaction to milk and it first showed up when she was three years old,' says her mum, Sylvia. 'She was on Ventolin syrup from the age of three, but her first hospital admission for an asthma attack was at the age of eight.'

Nicola, now sixteen, has spent much of her young life learning to manage her asthma, which at times has been very severe. 'It has been pretty grim,' admits Sylvia. 'We have to take her in to hospital quite regularly.' And every time Nicola is admitted to hospital, the whole family is affected. Says Sylvia: 'It is a strain on all of us. Her brothers and sisters all react in their own different ways. Her younger brother is always badly behaved when she goes into hospital.

For me the constant worry is – is she bad enough to take in to hospital? Shall I call the GP? Or the ambulance?'

Sylvia, a teacher, has worked part time: 'The hardest time was the years between aged ten and thirteen. You can't leave children when they are unwell, although my husband and friends have been tremendously supportive.'

TRIGGERS AND TREATMENTS

The main triggers for school-aged children's asthma are much the same as they are for adults (see page 25), covering the full range from cold air and exercise to pollution and pollen. But as a parent you may have to be on the alert for places or situations which bring on your child's symptoms.

About 60 per cent of schoolchildren with asthma are allergic to house dust mite droppings, and if your child comes into this category you may want to take the usual dust control measures (see page 113) such as damp dusting, minimal soft furnishing, mattress covers and fortnightly trips into the freezer for soft toys. Avoid putting allergic children in the lower half of bunk beds too.

Have you noticed that your child comes home from a friend's house feeling particularly wheezy? Perhaps that friend has pets who are to blame? If so, ask the friend to play at your house instead. Or maybe it's fumes from science experiments which are causing problems, or embarrassment about using an inhaler at school? If so, do have a word with teaching staff, who need to be well versed in what to do during an asthma attack: they may also like to read the National Asthma Campaign's literature for teachers. This recommends amongst other things that children should be allowed to carry their own inhalers at school. It's not good practice for asthma medicines to be locked away in the school office: in emergencies, inhalers need to be readily available, and children (although they may need discreet reminders) need to be able to take a puff of reliever medicines before or during sports.

And it is important that children with asthma do take part in school sports wherever possible. This helps keep them fit so that they are in better shape to resist infections and to cope with asthma. It also keeps them in the swing of things so that they don't feel left out at school.

Alternatively, if you have questions about your child's asthma, why not ring the National Asthma Campaign's Asthma Helpline (0345 010203) to speak to a qualified asthma nurse? Many of the 17,500 calls a year received by the Helpline are from parents needing reassurance about how to manage their child's asthma. (Calls are charged at local rates and the lines are open from 9 a.m. to 9 p.m. on weekdays.)

Conventional medical treatments for school-age children are much the same as treatments for adults, and most children with asthma will be prescribed inhaled relievers (plus preventers if necessary) by their doctors.

It is widely recognised that untreated asthma can limit growth in children. Naturally enough, though, many parents worry about the long-term effects of prescribing drugs to children. The most effective preventers include steroid drugs which children inhale – yet steroids have been given a pretty bad press in recent years. One 1991 study suggested that high doses of inhaled steroids can affect children's growth in the short term, although they will eventually grow to normal height. Yet there is also evidence that 'vigorous treatment early after diagnosis can improve the long-term outcome' (National Asthma Campaign report, *The Asthma Generation*). If this is true, parents may not feel so bad about dosing their children with steroids.

Alternatively, why not try one of the complementary or holistic treatments described in Chapter 7. These may help your child to cut down on his or her intake of conventional drugs, although it must be stressed that there is no substitute for modern drugs.

The positive side

And recently, things have been looking up for Nicola and her family. According to Sylvia:

> 'We have got her on to a management plan now and things are much better. Nicola now has a regime of regular treatment with a nebuliser and she is supposed to take peak flow readings regularly too. But the difficulty with teenagers is to get them to stick to their programme. Nicola does try to be very positive but she goes through phases where she just can't be bothered.
>
> 'We try to be positive too and we encourage her swimming – she got her gold recently – and her flute playing, which has helped her breathing no end. And she climbed to the top of Snowdon recently with her Venture group, and not by the easy route either!'

Sylvia is well aware that in a few years Nicola will be going away to college:

> 'There'll be no one there to run around after her checking that she's got her medicines, so she has to learn to stand on her own two feet. I do worry an awful lot about

her (she also has a very severe peanut allergy), but as she's getting older I am letting her take more control.

'I've got to hand over the responsibility to her. Even six months ago I was reminding her – have you taken this or that treatment? – but not any more. Although it is difficult, I have to let her go.'

CHAPTER 10

Asthma and Your Young Child

GROWING OUT OF ASTHMA?

The good news is that the younger children are when they first get asthma, the more likely it is that their symptoms will disappear by the time they are five, never to be seen again. It's not quite accurate to say that children 'grow out of asthma' although this does seem to be the case. Doctors prefer to talk about asthma going 'into remission', because once they have appeared then seemingly disappeared, asthma symptoms can reappear at any age.

Children who get asthma between the ages of three and five, as well as children who have allergy in their families, may well get over their symptoms by the time they are fourteen, although teenagers with asthma are likely to have symptoms throughout life.

The bad news is that there is much we still don't understand about asthma in small children. We can't measure the lung function of babies and young children with peak flow meters in the same way as we can with older children and adults. We don't even know why children under two years old become wheezy: it could be inflammation (as it is with adults), or it could be that little children's airways are extra sensitive in various other ways.

It does seem likely, however, that viruses such as the common cold are the main cause of asthma in the very young, as opposed to allergies which become more important as children grow older. (Breastfeeding can make babies more able to resist viral infections.) Indeed, some of the usual allergic triggers – house dust mites, pollen and moulds – don't seem to affect the under-fives, although some are allergic to furry animals and birds.

BY ANY OTHER NAME?

Doctors don't even agree on the terminology of asthma; a third of children will have wheezing episodes before they are five years old but will never have breathing problems again – and naturally enough doctors are reluctant to give them the label of asthma. All this means that doctors can be reluctant to diagnose small children as having asthma, and it may take quite a few trips to the surgery before you get to the bottom of your child's breathing problems – as Marion, Laura's mum, found to her cost:

> 'Laura was finally diagnosed at the age of four – but not before we had gone through recurrent bouts of what the doctors called bronchitis, croup and even pneumonia. On the night we thought she had croup we boiled so many kettles that we could hardly see Laura across the room. But the one thing I did clearly see was her throat which was being sucked in and out as she struggled to breathe.'

Once, Marion sat up all night as Laura coughed and vomited at intervals of about a minute: 'The doctor didn't come that night, as he thought it must be some kind of tummy bug. I was sitting there, holding a bowl and looking at her, thinking that she might not make it through the night. Eventually, it eased off – and we were left still not knowing it was asthma.'

At last, when Laura was four, the family doctor suggested she blow into a peak flow meter and the diagnosis of asthma was finally confirmed. 'It was a relief,' says Marion, 'because once we had a diagnosis, we knew what to do about treatment.'

Just a spoonful of sugar . . .

Laura was given four daily puffs of the preventer drug Intal, a non-steroid medicine which is good at defending against allergic and exercise-induced asthma. She was also prescribed salbutamol (Ventolin), the reliever most commonly used by children as well as adults. During an attack she would inhale salbutamol using a nebuliser. These days young children are only rarely given nebulisers because doctors prefer to give spacers which are less bulky and quicker to use when a child needs help in taking aerosol medication. Even babies can take inhaled medicines using a spacer attached to a face mask, and the spacer helps the drugs to reach the lungs in the correct quantities, rather than sticking in the child's throat or mouth.

Spacers can be decorated with stickers to make them more attractive to little children, and you can turn the business of taking medicine into a game by counting, or pretending the spacer is a trumpet.

Not all relievers, however, are effective for babies and children under eighteen months and some can even have a 'paradoxical' effect, narrowing the airways instead of opening them. Doctors tend to rely on trial and error to find the best reliever medicine and babies are often prescribed ipratropium (Atrovent) as an alternative to salbutamol or terbutaline.

And if non-steroid drugs like Intal aren't helping to prevent your child's asthma, your doctor may suggest a low-dose inhaled steroid instead. These may have minor side effects, like hoarseness of the voice and thrush in the mouth, but side effects can be cut down by using a spacer and doctors claim these drugs are safer for children than uncontrolled asthma.

If you are concerned about side effects, you may like to try one of the complementary or holistic therapies in addition to – but not instead of – your conventional treatments (see Chapter 7).

ON ATTACK ALERT

Asthma attacks are very variable in children, but for Laura they took a couple of days to develop. Marion would notice that her daughter was getting very tired. Then Laura would begin to sit in a strange position, arching her back so that her chest was stretched as much as possible: 'I'd just have to watch her carefully. Once, when an attack was building, I took her to the surgery. While we were waiting I noticed that she seemed very fidgety. When the doctor saw her he told me her twitchy movements were symptomatic of extreme oxygen starvation.'

Asthma attacks can be extremely alarming for children and parents alike, especially when children are very young, but the best advice is to try to stay calm so that you can follow a plan of action which you have agreed with your doctor or asthma nurse.

According to *Asthma News* (issue 38), the typical emergency plan will look like this:

- Sit your child upright – or hold a baby upright – as this position is safer than lying down.
- Give reliever medicine straight away, and repeat the dose (one puff into a spacer every 20–30 seconds for five minutes if necessary) until his or her breathing improves.
- Call the ambulance, or your doctor if he or she is nearer. (Remember to keep your follow-up appointment.)
- When attacks are slow to develop – and they can take anything from a few hours to a few days to build up – you may be able to give your child a short course of steroid tablets to head off the attack.

The slow and undramatic build-up of Laura's asthma attacks meant that Marion had difficulty in explaining to other people that her daughter was at risk:

> 'When she went to play at other children's houses I'm sure their parents thought I was just fussing. They could see a perfectly healthy-looking child, and I was trying to explain to them about the dangers of her asthma. It was hard to part with her sometimes, knowing that people might not be taking my warnings seriously.'

It's important to make sure that anyone who may be caring for your young child knows what to do in an emergency, whether they are friends, relatives or paid childminders. Childminders especially should have written instructions on using asthma medicines and warding off asthma attacks. Try to make sure there are no triggers in a carer's house, such as pets, which may cause problems, and check that adults won't be smoking anywhere near your child. Cigarette smoke is particularly harmful to small lungs and can set off asthma attacks.

MAKING PROGRESS

And in time, most parents get to grips with their child's asthma, learn exactly how to deal with it – and then sigh with relief as it eventually fades away. After a few bad years, Marion had got Laura's asthma well under control:

> 'The turning point was when we got our own peak flow meter to monitor her asthma. We marked her progress on a chart, morning and evening. When she was getting worse we could see a clear trend developing on the chart

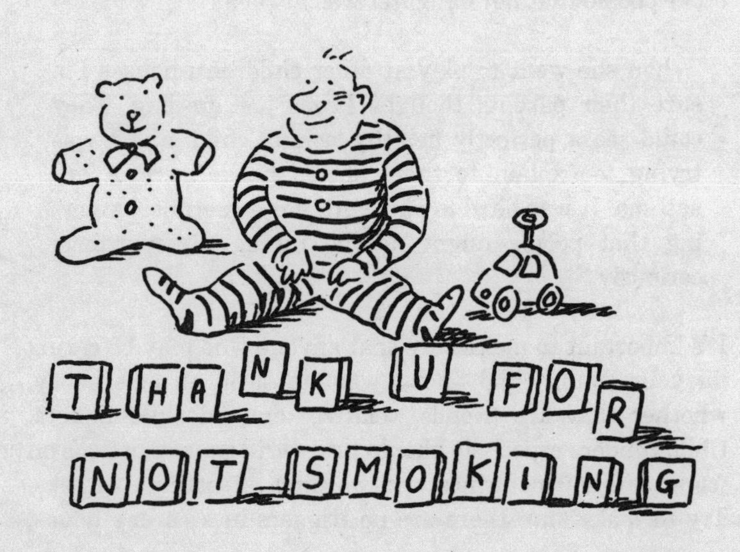

and we would step up the Intal and Ventolin. If her peak flow readings started to drop we would increase the doses. As a result of this monitoring, her asthma became pretty well manageable.'

From the age of eleven onwards, Laura seemed to 'grow out of' her severe asthma symptoms. Says Marion:

'She hasn't had an attack since she was twelve. At the back of my mind it is still there. I put it down on forms for school, and when she did work experience the doctor wrote that she must avoid fumes and dust.

'We still have a Ventolin inhaler at home and I remind her to take it when she stays with friends, but she's never had to use it. She still has a perpetual cough, but she's very active and good at sports. It doesn't hold her back at all. At last I feel we can talk about asthma in the past tense!'

CHAPTER 11

Keeping Fit with Asthma

SATURDAY NIGHT FEVER?

'I am pretty fit,' says Jeffrey, who is aged twenty-two, a student and a keen ballroom dancer. Talk to him a bit more and you'll realise this is a modest understatement: 'I like to go on outward bound type holidays,' he says. 'My favourites include mountaineering, canoeing, abseiling, potholing. Oh yes, and jumping off bridges into rivers – that's really good fun!'

Yet Jeffrey has quite severe asthma, requiring regular daily treatment with preventer and reliever medicines. How does he manage it? Because his asthma is well under control with a management plan agreed with his doctor, asthma doesn't stop him from taking part in any of the activities he so much enjoys. Only other people – ill-informed about asthma and anxious about asthma attacks – have tried to do that:

> 'Once I came down from a mountain and when we walked into the place where we were staying I started to wheeze. I got out my inhaler and said to the others, "Just give me a few minutes to get my breath back." The team leader said "Have you got asthma?" I said "Yes," and he said "Right, you're not going up any more

mountains." It meant that I missed out on climbing for the rest of the holiday which was very annoying.'

On another occasion, however, Jeffrey fared rather better:

'I take part in national ballroom dancing competitions, and after one jive competition I felt a bit wheezy so I took a puff from my inhaler. The coach saw me doing this and said that in future she would refuse to teach me the fast dances. Well, when she said that I went straight on to the dance floor and did the fastest jive possible!'

So what was the coach's reaction?

'Er, she backed down . . .' says Jeffrey.

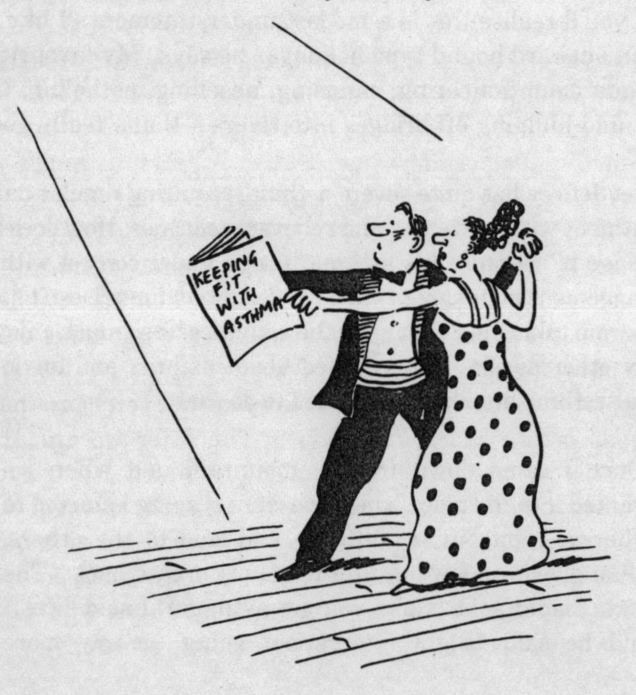

EXERCISE: THE ULTIMATE IN SELF HELP?

In fact, far from being a bar to taking exercise and doing sports, asthma is a very good reason for keeping as fit as possible. And when you think of those well-known athletes who have made it to the top in their chosen sport – they include Adrian Moorhouse, Ian Botham, Steve Ovett and Liz Hobbs – it's a fair bet that having asthma has made them all the more determined to succeed!

Exercise is good for everybody, and especially good for people with asthma. It keeps us in good shape both physically and mentally, toning muscles, strengthening our hearts and lungs, burning fat and contributing to our sense of confidence and well-being. In fact, of all the 'self-help' strategies we can call on to stay healthy, exercise is one of the most effective – as well as being cheap, safe and free from side effects!

Children in particular need to take part in vigorous games and sports. The hormones which their bodies must make so that they can grow are produced during exercise (as well as in sleep). Socially too, most children have a need to join in and to do well in the eyes of their peers. 'Wimp' is a damaging label for anyone to carry, and when uncontrolled asthma is the cause of a child being picked on, it is not only cruel but unnecessary.

Arguably, people with asthma can benefit even more than 'normal' people can from exercise. The fitter we are, the more able we are to fight off infections which can trigger asthma attacks. The more exercise we take, the stronger our lung muscles will be – and the more able we are to cope with breathing difficulties during attacks. Indeed, some doctors say that of their patients with asthma, those who take regular exercise feel better and report fewer problems.

Warm up, shape up

Having said all that, people with asthma do need to tackle the question of exercise with a little more care and forethought than usual. If you have 'exercise asthma', or exercise-induced asthma, running about – without a warm-up and without medication – can bring on exactly the symptoms of breathlessness, coughing and wheezing that you want to avoid.

There are several simple things you can do to make sure that you can enjoy exercise safely and without bringing on an attack. In their booklet *Exercise and Asthma* the National Asthma Campaign recommends that you do the following:

- Warm up before vigorous activities by making several thirty-second sprints over a period of five to ten minutes. This gives the lungs (as well as the rest of the body) the chance to adapt to the demands about to be put upon them.
- Take medication such as sodium chromoglycate (Intal or Cromogen) – a preventer which can be used 30 minutes before exercise – to prevent symptoms, or blue relievers taken 5–10 minutes before exercise.

Your choice of sport – and when you do it – can also help you keep asthma symptoms at bay. For instance, prolonged exercise which involves using your whole body, like running, makes more demands on the lungs than less prolonged, less strenuous exercise, like walking for instance.

And if you go for a long run on a frosty winter's day when the air is cold and dry, you are more likely to have problems than if you do some short sprints at a summertime athletics meeting. This is because you will be taking in a lot of air and quickly, so that the lining of your lungs loses moisture and they become more 'irritable'.

Swimming is very popular with people who have asthma – indeed, there are many swimming groups within the National Asthma Campaign – for the same reasons. The air around most indoor pools is warm and moist, just as your lungs like it to be, so that puffing up and down for length after length is going to make you fit and strong without putting your airways under additional strain. (Some children, however, find that chlorine can trigger an asthma attack.)

Puffed out

But if your symptoms are relatively mild, how do you know whether you have exercise-induced asthma – or whether you are just a bit puffed out after running around? It is important to get the answer to this right, because if your wheezing is a clue to a diagnosis of asthma, the right treatment can help you to enjoy exercise again without further problems.

Your doctor can check you out for asthma by giving you breathing tests (peak flow readings) when you arrive at the surgery and then again after you have taken some kind of exercise, such as running around the block for a few minutes. Some 80 per cent of people with asthma will have a fall in their peak flow reading within ten minutes after exercise. If a couple of puffs of reliever medicine then rapidly improves your breathing, this is another sign of asthma.

And even when asthma is particularly severe, the right kind of exercise and physical fitness can lead to achievements that put the rest of our couch-potato generation to shame.

Nicola, now sixteen, has been in and out of hospital with severe and chronic asthma all her life. 'She walks to school regularly to keep fit,' says her mother Sylvia, 'and she got her gold in swimming recently. She goes to Ventures too; she got to the top of Snowdon with them, not by the easy route either! I don't want her doing the peak assault however (in which a series of peaks are attempted), I would worry about that . . .'

Well, Sylvia, wouldn't we all?

CHAPTER 12

On Holiday with Asthma

WISH YOU WERE THERE?

You've worked hard all year and you deserve a break. The travel agents' windows are plastered with enticing offers: holidays in the sun; trips to exotic islands; visits to foreign cities. You think of days spent relaxing on the beach, enjoying delicious seafood, soaking up a different culture . . .

Then you think of asthma . . . What will happen if your breathing, or your child's, takes a turn for the worse? How will you be affected by the climate? By the air quality? By the food? You imagine yourself frantically looking for the hospital, trying to communicate with doctors in a foreign language. Will they have the drugs you need? And what about the expense of medical bills? According to Laura's mother:

> 'Laura's asthma was a major consideration when it came to planning holidays. Year after year we thought of going abroad – only to decide against it. What would we do if she had an asthma attack? How would we be able to get hold of a nebuliser, or would we be able to plug in our own? Her asthma was often triggered by

excitement – which is what holidays ought to offer after all. And we'd read an awful story about a little girl who'd had an attack while on a Greek island. She was given an emergency tracheotomy, which didn't help things at all . . .'

Worries like these are close to the top of the list for many of us with asthma in the family, but with sensible planning and forethought, there is no reason why your holiday snaps shouldn't be as interesting (or excruciating?) as anyone else's each year.

Good morning campers!

The key to success is making sure that your holiday destination will be good for you – in more ways than one. There is no single, ideal place for people with asthma to go, because we all experience asthma differently and find that different 'triggers' will set it off.

If pollen gets you going, then a camping holiday in midsummer is not going to do you an awful lot of good. Charles had a miserable time the last time he slept in his tent: 'It was stormy weather, which may have brought down pollen – or else polluted air – to ground level. I lay awake all night and all that I could think of was the next breath. It was really frightening.'

If, on the other hand, you are allergic to animals, then farm holidays and pony trekking are best left to other folk.

Air pollution may be the trigger which causes your problems, in which case check with your travel agent or the country's tourist office about the air quality at your destination. It's a safe bet that most big cities these days – particularly those surrounded by hills – are pretty polluted.

Staying ahead of the field

Those of us who are sensitive to pollen know that different plants, all flowering at different times of year, can be the source of trouble. Grass pollens, for instance, are a common trigger, and these reach their height in this country during the early months of summer.

So if you are going on holiday in the UK in summer – and school holidays may mean this is the only time you can go – it's worth looking out for holiday spots where pollen counts are lower, such as beaches with onshore breezes, or places up in the hills. Of course, the ideal way to avoid pollen altogether (not to mention the perils of pets) is to go for a cruise on an ocean liner – if you can afford it, that is!

And unfortunately for sun worshippers, grass pollen levels reach their peak on hot, sunny days, so you may be better off staying indoors with the windows closed, or keeping your car windows shut if you do go out (some modern cars have pollen filters). Mornings, when pollen is released, and evenings, when the 'pollen cloud' comes down to earth are the worst times. Damp cool days may not improve your tan, but they will cut down on the pollen count.

Alternatively, look in the local paper – or listen to the radio – to check the day's pollen forecast before you set out with bucket and spade. The pollen count is defined as the average number of pollen grains in each cubic metre of air, and daily checks and forecasts are made in many places across the country. If you want to be really efficient about it, you could write to the Pollen Research Unit at the University of North London (see Resources and Contacts). If you send them an SAE and information about where you want to go, they will let you know the likely pollen problems in advance. But be sure to contact them at least two months in advance of booking your holiday so that they can get the information to you on time.

A mite chilly?

Another way to avoid pollen is to take a winter holiday. An added bonus for skiers is that house dust mites don't survive above the snow line – which puts paid to another major asthma trigger. But if it's cold air which plays havoc with your lungs, the *piste* is obviously not for you!

As for that other common asthma trigger, the house dust mite, you might want to ask about whether your hotel or rented accommodation has synthetic pillows and duvets. If not, you could take your own, together with a mattress cover to fend off the worst effects of the dreaded mite.

Alternatively, head for the hills – where the mites don't

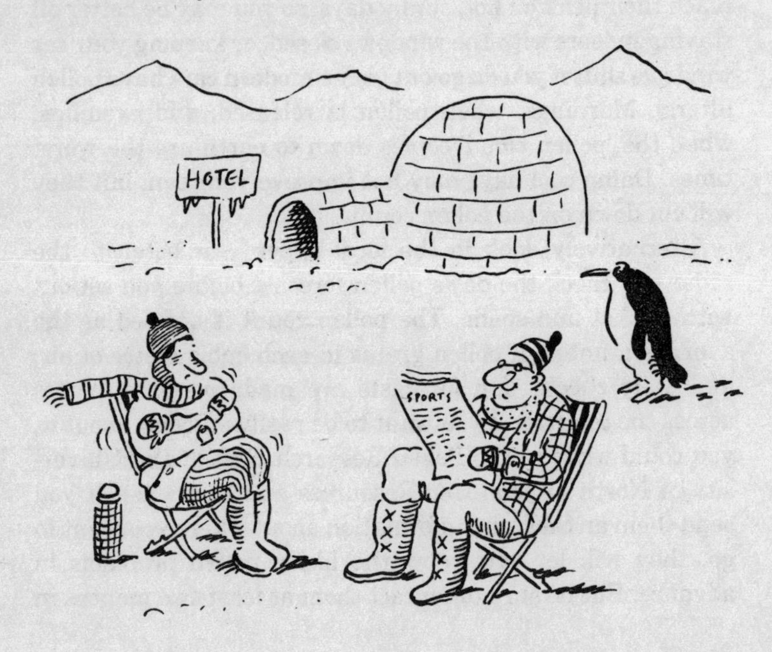

survive – or book a special low-dust room in a Swiss or Finnish resort. Tourist information offices should be able to tell you about European countries which offer these rooms to visitors, and at least one new initiative in the UK (see Resources section) means that low-allergen holiday homes will soon be available here.

And a few more tips regarding triggers: people whose asthma is made worse by mould spores might want to avoid autumn breaks, as this is the time when mould spores are at their peak. People who suffer after contact with pets would be wise to check that wherever they are planning to stay does not allow pets. Remember that the trigger carried by animals can stay in the environment for weeks after the pet has moved on.

BE PREPARED

Having chosen the best destination for your lungs, what else can you do to make sure that asthma doesn't limit the fun of your holiday? Most of the precautions recommended by doctors are plain common sense. For a start, why not pay a visit to your GP before setting off on holiday so that you can work out your own asthma management plan? He or she should outline which treatments you should take, and when, as well as how much you can increase them if you need to. A management plan and/or treatment adjustments before the holiday will usually mean you can go anywhere.

When it comes to packing, make sure you take enough medicines to last you through the trip – and then some more. Should you be unlucky enough to face flight delays or cancellations – or miss a flight – the last thing you need is the added stress of worrying about running out of medication. And pack your medicines as hand luggage to travel with you, so that the nightmare of suitcases going missing won't necessarily mean the end of your holiday plans.

The National Asthma Campaign recommend that you take your usual reliever and preventer medicines, some spare prescriptions, plus your asthma management plan and peak flow meter. For emergencies they also suggest you take an aerosol reliever inhaler (usually blue), plus steroid tablets (such as Prednisolone). Rotacaps and Spincaps (inhalers) may not function properly in hot, humid climates, and so a different type of inhaler may be appropriate.

If you use a nebuliser, say the National Asthma Campaign, who publish a special leaflet *Asthma and Holidays*, ask your travel agent what voltage is used in the country of your destination, and check that your nebuliser will work there (the manufacturer will be able to tell you for sure). Hand-pump and battery-operated nebulisers are also available. In an emergency they recommend using a disposable coffee cup as a mask or a spacer by making a hole in the bottom to fit over the inhaler mouthpiece.

Write down the names of your medicines before you leave home and then, if you can, get them translated into the language of your destination. Do the same with names and phone numbers of the hospital casualty and ambulance service nearest to where you are staying: holiday representatives or hotel staff should help you with this.

I'm Virgin; fly me?

Perhaps the greatest bonus of travelling to your holiday spot by air is that you're not likely to be stuck on board an airplane for more than a few hours at a stretch, which means the chances of an asthma attack several miles high are pretty slim.

However, very few airlines carry their own nebulisers on

board, with the exception of Virgin and Cathay Pacific. If this concerns you, check before you book your flight. Also make sure when you book that you get a seat which is well away from the smoking section. Better still, book with an airline which has banned smoking altogether.

BETTER SAFE

Chances are you will have a wonderful, asthma-free holiday. But chance being what it is, the one time you don't bother with medical insurance will be the one time you really need it. Private insurance really is a must for any country outside of the EC, and even within the EC you may have to pay the full cost of any medical care, although you can claim money back when you get home as long as you have filled in form E111 before you go.

And here is a practical tip from Jean Springett who wrote to *Asthma News* after deciding to take a holiday in France. Jean travels with a portable oxygen cylinder which she needs to use in places where the air is polluted. But how, while in France, could she get a large cylinder to replace her smaller one?

'My chemist suggested I get in touch with a chemist in Paris,' says Jean, 'who would supply oxygen to the hotel in which we were staying. This we did without difficulty.' The oxygen cost about £50, which Jean thought she could claim back when she got home using form E111. But not so; when she got back to the UK Jean discovered that E111 is for emergencies only, and she needed to fill in form E112, obtainable from the International Relations Unit (see Resources and Contacts).

Happy holidays!

CHAPTER 13

On the Home Front

In today's polluted and stressful world, wouldn't it be nice to think that there is at least one place – your home – where you can feel safe from whatever it is that causes asthma? But ironically, the more you strive to make your home into a warm and cosy haven, the more likely you are to be causing yourself problems.

For the modern centrally heated, freshly decorated, insulated and double-glazed home – with its much beloved family pet and cultivated garden – may be as much to blame for setting off your wheezing and coughing as any busy road or smoke stack outside.

HOUSE OF LITTLE HORRORS

Although the physicians of old (see Chapter 1) suspected that asthma was connected to breathing in house dust, it wasn't until the 1960s that scientists spotted the real culprit – a tiny creature called the house dust mite, or *Dermatophagoides Pteronyssinus*. This creature is truly hideous with its blind, tick-like body and spidery legs. (It is an arachnid, not an insect, and so belongs to the same family as ticks and spiders.)

And I don't know which of the many horrible aspects of the dust mite is the worst: that up to two million of them are likely to be living in your mattress alone? Or, that they live by eating the little bits of human skin that we all shed at the rate of one gram per day? Or, that it is the dung (faecal particles) of the mite which we breathe in when dust is disturbed that can cause an allergic reaction?

As if all that weren't bad enough, each of these little horrors produces twenty faecal particles for every day of their ten-week lifespan – during which time they also produce up to eighty eggs to make lots more little dust mites!

No matter how houseproud you are, it's almost certain that the dust mite lives in your home, colonising the dust that inevitably gathers in all carpets, fabrics, furnishings and bedding. Any new piece of furniture that you bring into the home will swiftly become colonised too.

But don't despair; the one saving grace of the dust mite is that at 0.3mm long, it is so small that you can't see it without a microscope. And there are simple steps you can take to combat its numbers – by controlling things like the temperature and humidity of your home.

'The best conditions for mite growth are to be found in sealed-up – and therefore humid – centrally heated homes,' says Jill Warner PhD, the National Asthma Campaign's Senior Research Fellow and Lecturer in Child Health at Southampton University Hospital, whose special area of research is the way young children can become sensitised to allergens in the first years of life. 'Where temperatures are around 25°C and humidity is about 80 per cent [which happens in some homes],' says Dr Warner, 'this is an ideal environment for mites to grow and breed.'

And where do mites like it best? In your bed, of course,

where the warmth and moisture of your body overnight – plus all those yummy skin scales – are just what little *Dermatophagoides* likes best! In drier homes, mites lay fewer eggs and die faster, which is why there are special asthma clinics in the Alps where the air is cold and dry.

BEATING THE BEASTIES

But how can you – apart from turning down the central heating and throwing open the windows – make your home as uncomfortable as possible for the dust mite without making it too uncomfortable for yourself? After all, few of us

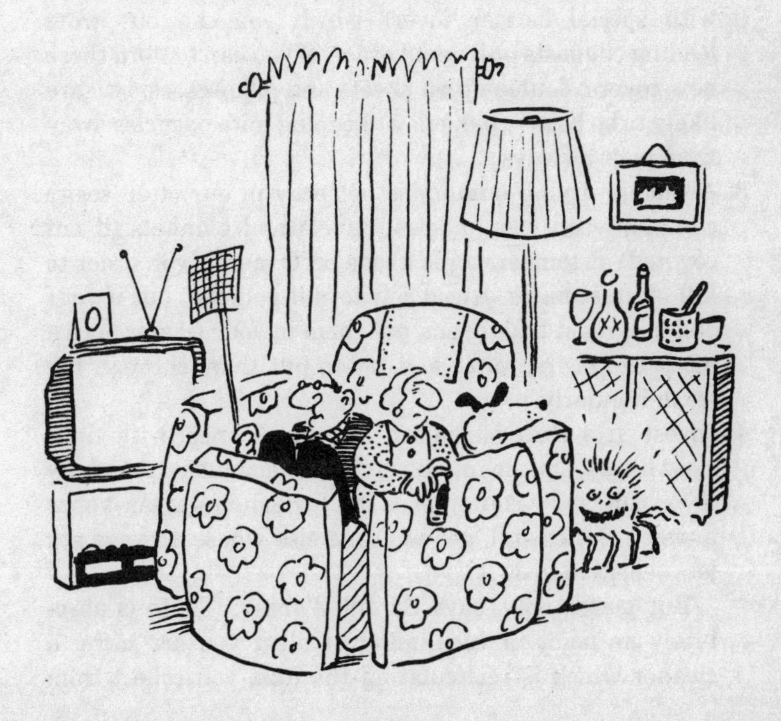

would want to go without carpets, curtains and cushioned furniture altogether, or give up the mattress on our beds.

Fear not: help is at hand with new techniques designed to reduce mite numbers without requiring you to live like a monk. Concentrating on the bedrooms and living room, Dr Jill Warner recommends that you try a combination of the following measures:

1. Get rid of as many mite havens as you can (i.e., carpet, curtains, soft furnishings), especially from your bedroom. But where you must have carpets, stick to short pile and preferably synthetic varieties.
2. Cover that mattress – as well as your pillows and duvet – with special barrier covers which you can buy from leading chemists or by mail order. If you can't afford these new covers, double up on sheets and pillowcases: two are likely to be better than one at keeping mite particles away from your airways.
3. Although drying laundry is not easy in our often soggy climate, wash your pillows, duvets and blankets (if not covered) at temperatures above 55°C monthly in order to kill off dust mites. Avoid soft toys if you can, but if your children must have them, put them in your freezer once a week to kill the mites and try to put them through the wash regularly.
4. Invest in a state-of-the-art vacuum cleaner, with first-class filters, and clean, clean, clean! Vacuum carpets daily if you can, and vacuum those soft furnishings at least once a week. Better still, get someone else whose airways are less sensitive to do it.

   But please note, says Dr Jill Warner: 'There is absolutely no point in vacuuming at all if you are using a cleaner which is recirculating the dust you collect from the surfaces back into the air – as is the case with many standard cleaners which are not fitted with filters to prevent re-emission of particles.'

Which brand of vacuum cleaner should you buy? Scientists are now testing various makes of cleaner to find out exactly which are best for mite control.

5. Cut down the humidity in your house if you can. Simple ways of doing this are to open windows during or after cooking, showering or having baths (unless you are allergic to pollen, in which case open windows only at night). Also try to dry laundry outside, rather than indoors and/or over radiators. Trials are currently underway in Denmark to see if better ventilation systems in our homes might help.
6. You might want to try one of the chemical mite killers, called acaricides, which are sprays and liquid treatments for carpets and soft furnishings. But a note of caution if you have children or are planning to become pregnant: these chemicals have yet to be fully tested for safety and should be used only under medical advice, and never on beds and pillows.
7. Chuck away that feather duster, as well as your soft dusting cloths, and dust surfaces with a damp cloth instead. Alternatively, use a vacuum attachment with your efficient new vacuum cleaner.

LETTING OUT STEAM

Another microscopic breathing hazard in your home is the tiny spores released into the air by the mould which often grows on damp surfaces. Like dust mites, mould spores are an allergen which can bring on all the symptoms of asthma.

And like dust mites too, mould spores are lurking in every home. However, only where damp has got a grip will mould grow in spots or patches – which can be blue, green, brown or black – ready to release more spores.

So how can you get rid of mould and its spores? Ideally, the answer is to get rid of any damp in your home. Sometimes damp is the result of some kind of leak: water may be seeping through your roof, rising from under your floor-boards or dripping from a leaky pipe. This usually calls for some kind of structural repair which will put an end to the damp problem.

But damp can also be caused on a day-to-day basis by too much condensation inside your home – whether it comes from cooking or from laundry or from the bath. In this case, try to prevent your house from becoming cold, using some kind of background heating such as storage heaters which will stop moist air from condensing on cold surfaces. Try to make sure the kitchen and/or bathroom is well ventilated, in order to let out any steam.

DIY DANGERS

The more you care about your home, the more likely you are to spend time trying to improve it. And that usually means using one of the range of solvent-based paints, varnishes, cleaning fluids, glues, damp-proof courses or chemical wood treatments which can have the unwelcome effect of irritating your airways – and even causing an asthma attack.

Common sense – and the instructions for using most of these products – will tell you how important it is to open the windows in the room where you are working. Better still, do the work outside. But if you have to work in an enclosed space, make sure you don't stay there for long without coming up for air.

Alternatively, it is now possible to buy a range of virtually solvent-free emulsion paints (see Resources and Contacts). You may also want to ask yourself: 'Is this job really necessary?' And if you decide it is, why not ask – or pay – someone else to do it for you?

Incidentally, clothes which have been dry-cleaned may also be releasing solvent vapours, so make sure they are dry when they get back to you and try to give them a good airing before wearing!

And if you want to know more about indoor pollutants, you can send for a free booklet from the Department of the Environment called *Good Air Quality in Your Home* (see Resources and Contacts).

The Building Research Establishment Advisory Service (BRE) also offers advice on air pollutants in houses, although you may have to pay for this advice. Contact the Building Research Establishment; their address and phone number can be found in the Resources section at the back of the book.

IN AN ENGLISH COUNTRY GARDEN

What better place to escape the fumes, the moulds, the mites and other asthma triggers than in your garden, that traditional English site of recreation and healthy exercise? Wrong. The classic English garden with its grassy lawn, hedges and border of trees may be beautiful to look at, but it is also a pollen and mould spore trap which could have been designed especially to aggravate your asthma.

But again, all is not lost for those of us with green fingers.

It is possible to have a garden which causes you the minimum allergic reaction by organising it carefully. Indeed, since 1993 the National Asthma Campaign have promoted the concept of the 'Low Allergen Garden' at the annual Chelsea Flower Show and have been rewarded with prizes for their efforts.

This kind of garden avoids wind-pollinated plants such as grasses and trees, as well as heavily scented and/or pollinated flowers – such as those from the daisy family. It also avoids hedges, which can trap large amounts of pollen and mould spores, and uses trellises to support climbing plants instead. Gravels are used instead of mulches (which release mould spores), and ground cover plants are encouraged to reduce weeding (which can mean breathing pollen at close quarters).

Without grasses, of course, you can't have a traditional lawn, but at the Chelsea Flower Show, the National Asthma Campaign Low Allergen Garden sported attractive but inexpensive paved areas, with potted plants at intervals.

And a note about timing your visits to – or work in – your low allergen garden. Dull damp days, or alternatively, early mornings, are best for people with allergies to pollen. But sunny days are best if you react to mould spores, which tend to be released in damper weather.

HOME SWEET HOME

But it's not all bad news for modern home owners. On a positive note, there is much about today's homes which can make life easier for people with asthma. That double glazing may be encouraging mites to breed if you don't open the windows (especially the bedroom windows) from time to time, but your windows can also shut out pollen clouds in summertime and mould spores in the autumn.

And central heating, while it too encourages mites, prevents asthma symptoms in those of us who start to wheeze if we go from a warm room to a cold one, or when we meet a gust of cold air.

There are also many encouraging developments in the design of new homes. The concept of the 'low allergen house' – a home built and furnished to improve the indoor environment and promote healthy living – is up and running in this country as well as in Europe (see Chapter 16). In short, the home of the future is a healthier home for us all.

CHAPTER 14

Asthma and Work

A STRANGE EPIDEMIC

Here is a cautionary tale of asthma caused – and asthma prevented – in the course of a modern day's work.

During the 1980s, the Spanish city of Barcelona suffered repeatedly from a mysterious epidemic. For seven years in a row, at particular times of the year, Barcelona's hospitals

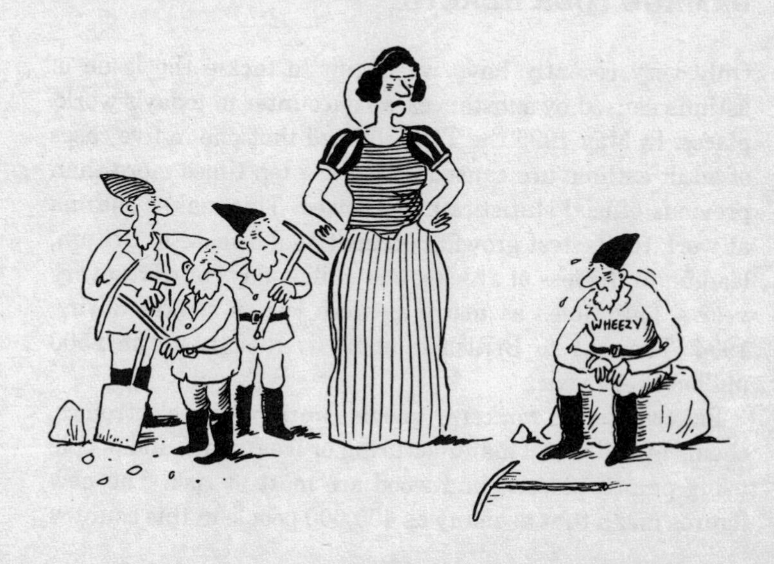

were awash with emergency cases of asthma. No one could work out what was going on – until a keen researcher spotted that a high proportion of the people struck by asthma lived near the city's harbour.

Investigators started to look at what could be happening at the harbour and discovered that on the days when the asthma epidemics reached their peak, cargoes of soya beans were being unloaded from ships docked at Barcelona. In due course they worked out that dust from the beans was being blown inland from the ships – triggering mass asthma attacks.

The solution? Simply by putting lids on the soya bean silos, Barcelona's asthma admissions were cut by twenty-five-fold.

WARNING: YOUR JOB COULD SERIOUSLY DAMAGE YOUR HEALTH

Only very recently have we begun to tackle the issue of asthma caused by substances we encounter in today's work-places. In May 1995 the TUC claimed that one in five cases of adult asthma are caused by work – ten times more than previous official statistics had allowed. This makes asthma at work the fastest growing occupational disease in Britain, leading to the loss of at least one million days of work every year – four times as many as were lost in strikes during 1994. The cost to British industry is thought to be £500 million every year.

Bakers, farm workers, people working in electronics, chemical and metal manufacturing or treatment, and people using paints, plastics and wood are most at risk. The new figures mean that as many as 400,000 people in this country are suffering from 'occupational asthma'.

Paul is one of them, as he told Rory O'Neill for the TUC's publication *Asthma at Work*. Paul worked for a refrigeration company and, as well as coming into contact with a range of foodstuffs including soya wheat and seafoods, ammonia would periodically leak from the cooling system. Paul had always been a superfit individual, involved in swimming, weight training and running, but within months of beginning work for this company he was hospitalised after a severe asthma attack: 'After three years of illness and taking large doses of steroids as well as numerous other drugs, my illness has become far worse,' he said. 'I have asthma, emphysema and bronchitis. But I also have other illnesses caused by the side effects of the drugs I have to take.'

Paul has now been awarded industrial injuries benefit for occupational asthma, but he says, there is no help for what has happened to the rest of his life: 'The symptoms they cannot treat you for are loss of confidence, depression, not seeing any future, not being able to do much physically . . . the list goes on. I have changed mentally as well as physically.'

RAISING AWARENESS

In 1994 the Health and Safety Executive (HSE) launched an awareness campaign for industry called 'Breathe Freely'. The aim of the campaign was to make employers and workers aware of the fact that – with the right kind of protection – most cases of occupational asthma need never arise in the first place.

The most dangerous jobs for developing this kind of

asthma are (in order): spray painting, chemical processing, working with plastics, baking bread, treating metal, working with laboratory animals and welding and soldering while assembling electronic equipment. People who work in these jobs are coming into contact with one or more of over 200 substances – called respiratory sensitisers – which can trigger asthma symptoms if inhaled. Chemicals found in paints and polyurethane foam are particularly dangerous, together with glues, resins and the fumes from soldering flux.

More surprising, perhaps, are the ill effects which come from what we may think of as healthy, outdoor jobs, such as farming, cutting wood and working with animals. The dust from flour, grain and hay can make occupational asthma a hazard for agricultural workers and bakers; wood dusts such as mahogany and western red cedar can also trigger symptoms – while animal urine and dander put another group of workers at risk of asthma.

In 1995 the TUC joined forces with the National Asthma Campaign to launch a new campaign against asthma at work. They put the emphasis firmly on prevention and on measures to protect people who already have asthma in the workplace. The TUC/National Asthma Campaign leaflet points out three ways to tackle exposure to triggers and sensitisers:

- Dangerous substances should be eliminated from workplaces or replaced by safe alternatives.
- Workers should be protected against dangerous substances which can't be eliminated by
  - using protective clothing and a mask;
  - isolating the danger from the worker;
  - extracting the hazard from the workplace.

- If neither of the above is possible, exposure should be reduced to the lowest possible level. The time spent in contact with a dangerous substance can be reduced, or less dangerous substances can be substituted.

A NINE TO FIVE PROBLEM?

So how do you know whether your asthma is 'occupational' or not? If your symptoms get worse during the working week, but improve when you have a period of time off, the chances are that something at work is damaging your health. The crucial period for developing occupational asthma is the first year or two in a new job. It is in this time that you are vulnerable to becoming 'sensitised' to a particular substance. In time, this sensitiser can 'switch on' the asthma process – which your body may be unable to switch off again.

The good news is that you can nip the whole process in the bud by recognising the sensitiser and taking steps to avoid it. The bad news is that – all too often – this can mean changing your job. But better to lose a job, perhaps, than suffer the years of increasingly poor health which can follow repeated exposure to the sensitiser.

In an ideal world, however, there doesn't have to be a conflict between your job and your health. By law (the Control of Substances Hazardous to Health Regulations 1994), employers must protect their workers from a number of dangerous substances and these include respiratory sensitisers. If they don't, legal action can be taken against them under the Health and Safety at Work Act, 1974. As Rory O'Neill puts it in *Asthma at Work*, 'the impact of our industrial policies and priorities is fuelling the dramatic increase in asthma numbers (yet) too little is being done to tackle this wholly preventable suffering.'

And because people with occupational asthma are classed as having a 'prescribed disease', you are eligible to claim compensation from the Department of Health and Social Security. And every year more and more people are claiming compensation for occupational asthma: in fact three times as many people are now claiming as did only six years ago.

Rory O'Neill recommends you take the following steps towards claiming compensation for occupational asthma:

- Go to your trade union representative who will refer you to a legal expert as soon as you experience symptoms of asthma.
- Claim as soon as your health is affected and make sure you are referred to a specialist to help gather the necessary evidence.
- Keep a record of your complaints (exposure to dust, fumes etc.), as well as of any safety information or training you have received.
- Keep a record of substances you are exposed to.
- Record details of safety measures at work, such as protective clothing.
- Keep a record of others in your workplace who have similar symptoms.
- Don't accept any offer of compensation without consulting your trade union rep and your lawyer.

It may not be as easy as putting a lid on the soya beans, but with occupational asthma the solution can be simple and good health can be restored to you.

CHAPTER 15

Asthma and Pollution

'I live by the sea,' says Joan, 'which means that when I go to a city I notice the pollution even more.' And in the summer months when sunlight turns exhaust fumes into dangerous low level ozone, the city becomes an environment which is almost too dangerous for Joan to visit:

> 'I went to London last June for a meeting. Unfortunately, I didn't take my nebuliser and – because of the exhaust fumes – I had a dreadful time. I sat up coughing and struggling for breath through the night, and the next day I felt terrible. I don't think people realise how awful you can feel after an asthma attack; you can't concentrate and everything is aching – especially your arms and legs – for lack of oxygen.'

TRUE COST OF THE CAR CULTURE?

Sadly, Joan's experience is becoming increasingly commonplace: as we near the end of the twentieth century, Britain's air pollution problem is getting worse. True, the infamous peasouper smogs of the 1950s have been banished from our cities together with the coal-burning fires and power stations

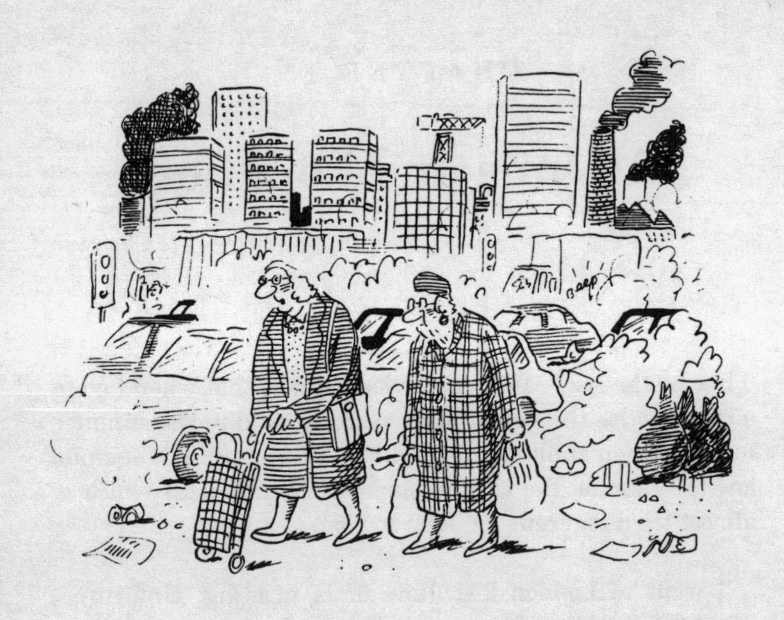

"JUST POPPING INSIDE FOR A SPOT OF FRESH AIR"

which caused them. But today, the threat of exhaust fumes has taken over with a vengeance.

Exhaust fume emissions have risen by 75 per cent since the 1980s – and with the numbers of vehicles on our roads set to increase by a massive 142 per cent before the year 2025 – they are likely to rise even further.

Pollution from vehicle exhausts is causing health problems to our whole population, but people with asthma, and children in particular, are especially at risk. People with asthma are experiencing breathing difficulties while stuck in traffic jams, while walking along busy roads, or simply, like Joan, when in town for a visit. And the long-term effects of breathing in these toxins, even at comparatively low levels, may also be very damaging.

There is, as yet, no proof that air pollution actually causes asthma in formerly healthy people, but many experts believe that it is to blame and that research now underway will prove this. Yet we do know for sure that air pollution can trigger asthma symptoms and can make the lungs more vulnerable to allergens – such as pollen – as well as viruses.

International research, from Europe to the USA, paints the same picture: there is a strong link between levels of ozone in the atmosphere and emergency hospital visits by children with asthma. Air pollution, even when it is below 'acceptable levels', reduces lung function. And it looks likely that levels of pollution which are too low to affect the lungs directly could still be causing damage – by making your airways sensitive to other airborne allergens which cause narrowing of the airways.

Children are especially at risk because, being small, their internal organs pick up higher concentrations of toxins. They also take in more air than adults in proportion to the size of their lungs. And since buggies have taken over from the old-fashioned high-sided prams, babies and toddlers are at just the right level to breathe in air polluted by cars and lorries.

WHERE BRITAIN LAGS BEHIND

Yet despite the dangers, Britain lags so far behind other comparable countries when it comes to monitoring air pollution that Friends of the Earth filed a complaint with the EC Commission in 1993. Japan has over 2,000 sites for monitoring air pollution; the Netherlands and Spain have around

200. In Britain, we have only thirteen Department of the Environment sites to measure sulphur dioxide and particulate levels. According to a Friends of the Earth briefing, 'government sites are badly located. EC legislation requires nitrogen dioxide monitoring in streets with heavy traffic, whereas too many government sites are in pedestrian precincts or up back alleys.'

What can you do about it? In cities today it is commonplace to see people – especially cyclists – breathing through masks in the hope of keeping the worst effects of pollution at bay. A mask with an activated carbon filter may be of help, but masks have not been clinically tested and there is no proof that they protect you from pollutants like sulphur dioxide, nitrogen dioxide or particulates from diesel fuel.

If you ring the Department of Environment Pollution Helpline (free on 0800 556677) you can find out when and where air pollution is high, thus giving you the option of staying indoors (or at least avoiding vigorous exercise) for the day.

If you have to go out, breathing through a scarf on cold days will help to warm the air before it gets to your lungs and may reduce wheezing. Local radio stations and newspapers sometimes carry air quality forecasts to give you up-to-date local information too.

The National Asthma Campaign in their booklet *Asthma and the Environment* also recommends that you stay in control of your asthma by monitoring your own peak flow performance and intake of reliever medicines. At times of high pollution your doctor may also suggest that you increase your treatments with preventer and reliever medicines until some days after the air quality has improved.

These are all helpful short-term measures, but surely in the long term there has to be a better way than taking extra medicines or staying indoors. Why should people with asthma be subject to a kind of curfew in order to allow drivers of cars and lorries free rein on the roads?

What we really need is a radical change in our transport policies so that public transport gets more support and the car becomes a less attractive option. If you feel strongly that our current policies are damaging to health, why not write to your local MP and your local and national newspapers, or join a group such as Friends of the Earth or Greenpeace, to protest about levels of air pollution? You could also contact your local National Asthma Campaign branch and encourage them to hold meetings on air pollution.

If it helps you or your children to breathe more freely, it's got to be worth a try.

WARNING: THESE POLLUTANTS CAN SERIOUSLY DAMAGE YOUR LUNGS (*Asthma News* issue 36)

- **Nitrogen dioxide (NO_2)** Although there is some disagreement about how dangerous NO_2 may be for people with asthma, NO_2 stops the tiny hairs which line the lungs (cilia) from doing their job of clearing out mucus and dirt. This means that pollutants can stay in your lungs, clogging your airways and making you more vulnerable to infections. Nitrogen dioxide pollution went up by a half during the 1980s.

  NO_2 is not only a pollutant in vehicle exhausts, however: even higher levels are found inside homes which use gas cookers and gas fires.
- **Pavement level ozone** When sunlight hits nitrogen dioxide it makes ozone which reacts with a multitude of other pollutants to create photochemical smog. Pavement

level ozone also inflames your airways, reduces the ability of your lungs to work properly and reduces your resistance to allergies. It is especially a problem in summer when sunlight is at its brightest.

And despite its name, pavement level ozone may not be at its worst on city streets: highest concentrations are often found in country areas downwind of polluted cities. It is a serious health risk to some people with asthma, especially children.

- **Sulphur dioxide (SO_2)** This pollutant comes from the burning of coal – mostly in power stations – and levels have gone down significantly since the Clean Air Act of 1956. But SO_2 can cause wheezing if you breathe it in while taking exercise, and in the long term it may inflame your airways and worsen the symptoms of asthma.
- **Particulates** As the name suggests, these are small particles of soot or dust which come mostly from diesel vehicles. When particulates get into the lungs they can cause a worsening of symptoms in people with asthma.

CHANGES IN THE AIR?

Under former Transport Minister Dr Brian Mawhinney (previously the Health Minister), the government began to make some constructive noises about car pollution. Dr Mawhinney is known to be particularly concerned about the link between asthma levels and rising pollution. He knows that in the big smog of 1991, 150 people died in London alone. Recently he conceded that Britain is running out of fresh air (*Guardian* 28/2/95). At least 20 million people are inhaling polluted air daily. Manchester, Glasgow and Cambridge exceed EU limits on air pollution while another thirty-seven cities come close to breaching the directive.

At the end of 1994 he announced that he wanted 'to take polluting vehicles off the streets' and set up a 'blitz' on polluting vehicles in our cities. In the event, some 5,000 vehicles were found to be below the MOT emission test standards – but that leaves about five million more polluting vehicles yet to be tackled.

In 1995 Dr Mawhinney moved a little further down the road towards cutting car pollution. In February he announced tighter MOT test standards with fourteen days (as opposed to twenty-eight) to repair offending vehicles, with fines of up to £2500 on motorists who neglect to service their cars – plus extra resources to extend the 'blitz' to twenty-three major cities and towns.

Can it be that successive governments' commitment to 'the great car economy' (as Mrs Thatcher put it), is shifting towards a different kind of transport policy? All of us who are concerned about asthma fervently hope so.

CHAPTER 16

Asthma in the Future

THINGS HAVE IMPROVED A LOT

Talk to anyone with asthma, and chances are they will tell you how much things have improved in recent decades. Janet is forty-three now:

> 'Things were dreadful for people with asthma when I was a child. There were times when I could barely walk to school and my father had to carry me upstairs to bed. My parents didn't understand it and doctors weren't sure what it was all about.
>
> 'There were all sorts of psychological theories: was it stress? Was it an over-anxious mother? My mother thought it was her fault – but then as mothers, we do take on any guilt that's going. Very little treatment was given: I had an inhaler device, but the doctors were reluctant to give it to me in case it became "habit forming".
>
> 'The breakthrough came with the new generation of drugs, but I wasn't sure how to use them properly. At college I had injections to stimulate my adrenal glands. It was all very haphazard. No one ever took me aside and said "this is how you manage your asthma" – until about ten years ago.'

Jeffrey is twenty-two and he recalls his mother having breathing difficulties when he was a child but nobody seemed to know why or what to do about it: 'I remember my mum having to stick her head out of the window at home in an attempt to breathe more easily. It was never diagnosed as asthma, so she had no treatment.'

Joan is seventy-one; she has had asthma all her life and has watched her children and grandchildren growing up with this condition. But asthma in Joan's childhood was a very different story from asthma today:

> 'I missed years of school, and was only able to go to university on a part-time basis. Things have changed a lot in recent years. Even five years ago a young mother was likely to be quite panicked by a diagnosis of asthma in her child. Nowadays she will know about asthma and be able to cope. These days there's nothing to stop people with asthma doing anything they want to.'

NO SMOKE WITHOUT FIRE

So can we expect to see even more improvements in our understanding and care of asthma in the future? And what are these improvements likely to be? There are positive changes ahead, predicts Dr Donald Lane, Chairman of the UK Task Force on Asthma and Consultant Physician at Oxford's Churchill Hospital.

As he told *Asthma News* (August 94) recently, the old-fashioned view of asthma as a single condition is on the way out, while the concept of asthma as a syndrome or 'set of symptoms' is winning ground. This will help doctors to develop more specialised treatments and to suit medicines to individual symptoms more effectively.

Dr Martyn Partridge, Chief Medical Adviser to the National Asthma Campaign and Consultant Chest Physician at Whipp's Cross Hospital in London, echoes this view:

> 'In ten years' time we'll still be using the same medicines, i.e. inhaled steroids, but we will be better at targeting these drugs to the needs of individuals. We'll also be developing other medicines which may halt part of the inflammatory process. Later on we may come to understand more about how the whole cascade of inflammation starts – and be able to switch it off.'

And in another decade or two, believes Dr Partridge, we will know more about what activates asthma in the first place: 'It could be that we will be offering pre-conceptual counselling for mothers-to-be whose children may be at risk.'

Crucial to all this is understanding the genetic aspects of asthma. We know that asthma and other allergic diseases may be an inherited tendency; what we still need to find out is why more and more people are now having this tendency activated – causing more and more asthma.

SAFEGUARDING FUTURE GENERATIONS

All in all, this is a hopeful picture, holding out the possibility that we may be able to prevent future generations from developing asthma while they are newborns or still in the womb. Prevention – the current buzzword right across the health spectrum – could mean improving the air we breathe, not only in our cities but in our homes. We know that smoking in pregnancy makes children more likely to develop asthma, but only more research will tell us how other factors like food or pollution or our home environment may be putting future generations at risk.

Another kind of prevention, and one which many people already rely on, means stopping asthma from developing or worsening by using medicines (preventers), or by avoiding allergens. And there is plenty of research going on in this field too.

At Southampton University, Dr Jill Warner and her team of scientists are studying how our home environment affects the development of asthma and allergies, and whether this process can be delayed or prevented. So far Dr Warner has concentrated on the house dust mite and how it can cause allergies to develop when we are babies – and even before we are born. In the process she is becoming a world expert in vacuum cleaners and mattress covers!

A BREATH OF FRESH AIR

Linking up with Dr Warner's work is the concept of the Low Allergen House. Researchers in this country are now building on the advances made by the innovative 'Healthy Housing Project' at Laerkbo in Denmark. The Danes showed how our modern indoor climate – which more often than not is centrally heated and double-glazed – is positively heaven for the house dust mite, but positively hell for people with asthma.

Given that up to 80 per cent of adults with asthma are allergic to mites (another 40 per cent react to animal allergens), it made perfect sense to change that home climate. Engineers and architects got together with doctors to examine the construction of houses, and the result was a unique collection of 110 houses near Aarhus on the east coast of Jutland.

The Laerkbo houses were fitted with special ventilation systems to make sure that plenty of fresh, pollen-filtered air circulated through the rooms, keeping down humidity and discouraging mites from breeding. Pets were strictly kept out; kitchen furniture was made of wood to cut down on formaldehyde fumes; all paints were either water-based or silicate-based – again to reduce irritating fumes.

Families who moved into the homes found not only that the asthma sufferers amongst them felt much better but that the design of the houses seemed to increase everyone's well-being all round!

In 1994, the UK 'National Asthma Campaign Low Allergen House' was launched at the FutureWorld Exhibition in Milton Keynes. It had many of the qualities of the Laerkbo houses but it also showed how any house can draw on these ideas to cut down on indoor allergens. Again, ventilation was all important, with air being filtered, heated and circulated through ducts to all the rooms. Because this air is dry and fresh it spells death to mites.

Heating was at skirting board level to avoid the dust turbulence created by conventional radiators, while vacuuming was done through an inbuilt vacuuming system which takes dust directly from the house into an outside bin. Instead of curtains, the house had blinds; instead of carpets it had lino; instead of chipboard it used polished wood.

The National Asthma Campaign Low Allergen House incorporated ideas from the Low Allergen Garden (exhibited at Chelsea Flower Show) which used gravel mulches and ground cover to defeat weeds, paved terracing instead of lawns and trellises rather than hedges.

RESEARCH: MAKING PROGRESS THROUGH SCIENCE

As well as practical innovations like these, a great deal of work is also going on around the country into identifying the causes of asthma and how it may be treated in the future. Millions of pounds are being spent on looking at the lungs themselves to find better treatments. Other research on the environment is taking place, focusing on the things which trigger asthma symptoms such as smoking, chemicals in the workplace, vehicle exhaust emissions and other forms of air pollution.

Scientists are also looking into the safety and efficacy of modern medicines and how we care for people with asthma. One London study is looking at evidence that the over-use of beta agonist inhalers (these are the reliever drugs including Ventolin and Bricanyl) may be making asthma symptoms worse instead of better.

If the researchers do find that high doses of beta agonists are working against steroid treatments used to counter inflammation in the lungs, this could provide one reason why asthma is on the increase these days.

Other studies are looking at how asthma affects the population, comparing wheezing in different groups of children, for instance. The hope is that if we can identify asthma early on we could more effectively prevent it from developing.

One paediatrician, Professor Mike Silverman of Leicester University, has been funded by the National Asthma Campaign to map out the different patterns of wheezing in pre-school children. As yet we don't even know whether wheezy children have inflamed lungs or not, but Professor Silverman has developed a method of measuring inflammation in children's lungs by asking them to inhale a fine spray of salt water and analysing the sputum (phlegm) they produce. If he can discover more about the causes of childhood asthma this way, we may be able to produce more effective treatments for children in the future.

A SHIFT IN THE BALANCE

This is of course only a brief summary of the complex and in-depth scientific investigation currently going on into asthma in this country. But what of our role in tackling asthma – in ourselves, in our families, in our communities?

More and more as we reach the end of this century, people are grasping the wide-ranging implications of the apparently simple principle of self help. The days when doctors knew best and patients asked no questions have gone. Today, doctors and patients alike agree on the vital importance of good information, communication and cooperation when it comes to health. Doctors like Martyn Partridge see that this balance is going to shift even further in the future:

> 'It's going to be all about contracts between doctors and patients. Doctors will be saying "I'll be available for you to ring up and to answer your queries, and in return you will let me know how you are getting on with the drugs I have prescribed." It's no good having good drugs if they are not used properly. Our health professionals need to be well organised and well funded, while patients need to be able to express their fears and concerns.'

But will we still be relying on preventer and reliever drugs to control asthma symptoms in decades to come, or will we be tackling the root causes of this disease? 'Regrettably, for the time being,' says Dr Partridge 'a lot of people with asthma are only going to be able to lead normal lives by taking medicines.' He recognises that many of us are not entirely happy with that scenario:

> 'Most people aren't very impressed by drugs – although the current drugs are first class and have transformed the treatment of asthma in the past twenty or thirty years – and we do need to pay attention to our environment.
>
> 'Why has asthma increased so rapidly in recent years? If it has been environmental there may be a chance of changing that back. But studies into this issue are incredibly expensive and the pharmaceutical companies won't necessarily pay for the research, so all of us who believe this is an important issue need to do our bit to fund that research and to encourage the government and others to do likewise.'

HELPING OURSELVES TO HEALTH

So who is going to pay for research into possible environmental causes of asthma? In these days of minimal government funding for health care, we are back to the principle of self help.

Self help groups have sprung up across the Western world in recent decades for a wide range of medical problems. People join them looking for support, information and because they want to take control of their own health. They also join to support research, and asthma has been no exception.

The main UK asthma charity is the National Asthma

Campaign which was formed out of two smaller charities in 1990. Since then its members have raised millions of pounds for research – as well as setting up around 200 local branches. (For other National Asthma Campaign services, see Resources section).

Janet, whose story begins this book, became involved in fundraising for asthma research some years ago – at about the same time that she began to get to grips with her asthma – and she is now an active member of the National Asthma Campaign. So let's allow her to have the last word:

> 'When I first developed asthma I was so ignorant of the basic medication. I felt powerless to intervene and I wasn't facing what this disease is; I was denying it. But then I had a serious asthma attack: I thought I was going to die and I promised myself – if I get through this, things are going to change.
>
> 'I did change my attitude and since then things have been dramatically different. I am more in control now and I have confidence in tackling my asthma. If I have any concerns I can contact my local asthma clinic; there is so much more known about asthma now.
>
> 'The old stigma is going. I'm a teacher and I take my inhaler into lessons and explain all about it to the children. Quite often they will say: "Oh yes, my sister has one too." It's all much more accepted now.
>
> 'Physical activities hold no more terrors for me either; I have my medicines as back-up. And I also take care of myself, using relaxation techniques. I'm trying aromatherapy massage at the moment, which is wonderful for reducing stress and keeping me healthy. I try to be sensible about my diet too. I can see my way through it all – and I've got back my peace of mind.'

Resources and Contacts

GENERAL BOOKS

Living with Asthma and Hay Fever, John Donaldson (Penguin, 1994).
Asthma at Your Fingertips, Mark Levy *et al.* (Class Publications, 1993).
Conquering Asthma: An Illustrated Guide to Understanding and Self-Care for Adults and Children, Peter J. Barnes and Michael T. Woodhouse (Manson Publishing, 1994).

OCCUPATIONAL ASTHMA

Asthma at Work, Rory O'Neill. Published by the TUC and Sheffield Occupational Health Project, 1995.
Preventing Asthma at Work: How to Control Respiratory Sensitisers, HSE Books, PO Box 1999, Sudbury, Suffolk CO10 6FS (£6.25).

ASTHMA AND THE ENVIRONMENT

Friends of the Earth and Greenpeace each produce their own literature on this subject.

Friends of the Earth,
26/28 Underwood Street,
London N1 7JQ

Greenpeace,
Canonbury Villas,
London N1 2PN

Good Air Quality in Your Home, A free leaflet from the Department of the Environment. Orders can be faxed on 0181 533 7700.

DoE Distribution Centre,
PO Box 151,
London E15 2HF

The Building Research Establishment produces a range of leaflets about substances like formaldehyde used in building materials.

BRE Bookshop,
Building Research Establishment,
Garston,
Watford WD2 7JR
Tel: 01923 664444

The Healthy House is a mail-order business providing products for people with allergies, asthma and other disorders.

The Healthy House,
Cold Harbour,
Ruscombe,
Stroud,
Glos GL6 6DA

Tel: 01453 752216.
Fax: 01453 753533.

Pollen Research Unit,
University of North London,
166–220 Holloway Road,
London N7 8DB

There is also an Environment Pollution Helpline: free on 0800 556677.

ASTHMA AND SMOKING

Action on Smoking and Health (ASH) provides information about passive smoking and tobacco smoke in your environment. ASH has launched the Breathing Space campaign, which aims to convince shops, banks, restaurants and so on to introduce smoke-free areas in our public spaces. *Passive Smoking: Questions and Answers* is a free leaflet from ASH.

ASH,
109 Gloucester Place,
London W1H 3PH

ASTHMA AND HOLIDAYS

Form E112 is obtainable from:

International Relations Unit,
Room 318,
Hannibal House,
London SE1 6TE

Health Advice for Travellers: a free leaflet from the Department of Health (including form E111 for free or reduced-cost emergency medical treatment in EC countries). Order it by phoning (free) the Health Literature Line on 01800 555777.

The Old Chapel House is – as far as we know – Britain's first holiday B and B hotel dedicated to people with severe asthma. Overlooking the sea, it is designed and built to be dust- and allergen-free, with 24-hour medical attention available.

Edward Willis,
Old Chapel House,
12 East Terrace,
Budleigh Salterton,
Devon EX9 6PG

See below for holiday projects run by the National Asthma Campaign. There is also a leaflet available from the NAC, *Asthma and Holidays*.

THE NATIONAL ASTHMA CAMPAIGN

The National Asthma Campaign,
Providence House,
Providence Place,
London N1 ONT
Tel: 0171 226 2260
Asthma Helpline: 0345 010203

The National Asthma Campaign represents the interests of people with asthma, actively campaigning for a better deal. It spends more on research into asthma than any other non-commercial concern, including the government, as well as offering education, support and advice about asthma. The National Asthma Campaign offers a wide range of services, summarised below:

Information booklets

The National Asthma Campaign publishes twelve information booklets designed to answer your queries on various aspects of asthma:

1a. Take Control of Asthma
1b. Asthma in the Under Fives
2. Spacers and Nebulisers
3. Exercise and Asthma
4. Asthma at School: A Teacher's Guide
5. Asthma and Holidays
6. Asthma and Pregnancy
7. Self-Management and Peak Flow Measurement
8. Asthma at Work: Are You Eligible for Compensation?
9. Hayfever
10. Steroid Treatment for Asthma
11. Asthma and the Environment

Asthma helpline

The National Asthma Campaign Helpline (Tel: 0345 010203, Mon-Fri, 9 a.m., to 9 p.m.) is staffed by specialist asthma nurses. Offering practical advice, emotional support and information it receives over 17,000 calls a year, many from parents or people with asthma themselves.

Junior asthma club

The National Asthma Campaign's club for children aged between four and twelve has round 4,000 members and publishes a magazine, *A for Asthma*, every term.

Local branches

There are some 160 branches of the National Asthma Campaign in Britain, all of which are run by volunteers. They organise regular meetings and may invite expert speakers as well as offering contact and support.

School pack and video

The National Asthma Campaign publishes packs designed for primary and secondary schools. The packs include materials to help teachers deal with asthma in school, plus information for pupils about asthma.

The twelve-minute video for teachers and school nurses is called 'Every Little Breath', and it is free on loan, or costs £5 to buy. The National Asthma Campaign also provides pupils with School Cards which explain their medication to teachers. Teachers may also be interested in the National Asthma Campaign's School Asthma Policy, adopted by many schools across the country.

Holiday projects

The National Asthma Campaign and National Eczema Society ran six joint holiday projects in 1994 and are hoping to expand their programme in the future.

Asian language videos

The National Asthma Campaign provides information videos in five Asian languages which are available on loan.

Quarterly magazine

Asthma News is the quarterly magazine of the National Asthma Campaign.

Video
'Getting your Breath Back; understanding asthma' is a forty-minute practical video guide to asthma for sufferers and their carers, £11.99 from the National Asthma Campaign.

SCHOOLS

Pilgrims' School in Seaford, East Sussex is a small boarding school and the only one of its kind in the UK dedicated to children from aged nine upwards with chronic asthma or eczema.

COMPLEMENTARY MEDICINE

General advice
British Holistic Medical Association,
179 Gloucester Place,
London NW1 6DX

Council for Complementary and Alternative Medicine,
179 Gloucester Place,
London NW1 6DX

Institute for Complementary Medicine,
PO Box 194
London SE14 1QZ

Research Council for Complementary Medicine,
60 Great Ormond Street,
London WC1N 3JF

101 Clinic and Good Health Company,
101 Seymour Place,
London W1H 5TG

Publications

Guide to Asthma and Eczema: Possible Causes and Likely Treatments, published by What Doctors Don't Tell You. Includes information about side effects of conventional drug treatments, plus suggestions for alternative treatments.

What Doctors Don't Tell You,
4 Wallace Road,
London W1
Tel: 0171 354 4592

Acupressure

The Shiatsu Society,
Foxcote,
Wokingham,
Berkshire RG11 3PG

Acupuncture

Acupuncture Association and Register,
34 Alderney Street,
London SW1V 4EU
Tel: 0171 834 1012

Aromatherapy

International Federation of Aromatherapists,
Dept of Continuing Education,
Royal Masonic Hospital,
London W6 OTN

Herbalism
National Institute of Medical Herbalists,
9 Palace Gate,
Exeter EX1 1JA

Homeopathy
British Homeopathic Association,
27a Devonshire Street,
London W1N 1RJ

Society of Homeopaths,
2 Artizan Road,
Northampton NN1 4HU

Reflexology
Reflexologists' Society,
44 Derby Hill, Forest Hill,
London SE23 3YD

INTERNATIONAL ADDRESSES

Australia
Asthma Foundation of Queensland
51 Ballow Street,
Fortitude Valley 4006

Asthma Foundation of Northern Territories
PO Box 40456,
Casuara,
N.T. 0811

Asthma Foundation of South Australia
341 Halifax Street,
Adelaide,
S.A. 5000

Asthma Foundation of New South Wales
Unit 1, Garden Mews,
82–86 Pacific Highway,
St Leonard's,
N.S.W. 2065

Asthma Foundation of Tasmania
Hampden House,
82 Hampden Road,
Battery Point,
Hobart,
Tasmania 7004

Asthma Foundation of Victoria
101 Princess Street,
Kew 3101,
Victoria

Asthma Foundation of Western Australia
61 Heytesbury Rd,
Subiaco,
W.A. 6008

Canada
Canadian Lung Association,
75 Albert Street,
908 Ottawa,
Ontario

Ireland
Asthma Society of Ireland,
24 Anglesea Street,
Dublin 2

New Zealand
Asthma Society of New Zealand,
PO Box 1459,
Wellington

USA
American Lung Association,
1740 Broadway,
New York

National Asthma Campaign Asthma Manifesto

Asthma remains a major challenge to all health professionals. It continues to cause considerable suffering and even death, despite the existence of effective treatments.

Shortfalls in healthcare, poor communication between patients and doctors and the failure of emergency services to respond quickly in cases of asthma are among the target areas for improvement highlighted in the National Asthma Campaign's Asthma Manifesto.

The Manifesto was launched during the 1993 Asthma Week and aims to draw the attention of the government and others to the needs of people with asthma and to raise the standard of care available.

Under the guidance of Dr Martyn Partridge, a team of doctors and nurses worked with patients to draw up a list of rights for people with asthma. In terms of healthcare provision, people with asthma have the right to expect the best possible care given according to nationally agreed guidelines by experienced and committed professionals.

GOOD COMMUNICATION

People with asthma have the right to expect:

- Written and verbal advice about their asthma clearly stating what action to take if their asthma worsens.
- The opportunity to express their expectations of treatment, their fears about the condition and their prescribed medications.
- To be made aware of sources of additional information and support such as the National Asthma Campaign.

IN PARTNERSHIP WITH THEIR DOCTOR OR NURSE

People with asthma have the right to:

- Select the best inhaler device for them.
- Monitor their own condition with a peak flow meter.
- Control their asthma by following an agreed self-management plan.

FROM THEIR GENERAL PRACTICE

People with asthma have the right to expect:

- General practices to adopt agreed policies for the management of asthma.
- Specially trained health professionals to review their asthma management.

AT HOSPITAL

People with asthma have the right to expect:

- Referral to a hospital specialist whenever necessary.
- To be seen by, or be admitted under the care of, a Consultant in Respiratory Medicine. Children should be seen by a Consultant Paediatrician with expertise in asthma.
- Effective communication between hospital doctors and their GP.

IN AN EMERGENCY

People with asthma have the right to expect:

- Their calls for help to be treated as urgent by all health professionals.
- A swift response by an ambulance which is staffed with trained paramedics and equipped with oxygen and nebulisers.
- On arrival in hospital to be given priority in the triage system.
- A follow-up appointment in a hospital asthma clinic or in their local practice.
- Prompt communication between Accident and Emergency and the local practice.

The manifesto also covers important issues such as asthma in the workplace, what children with asthma should expect at school and wider rights regarding liaison with insurance companies and consumer rights. The National Asthma Campaign also believes that the government needs to demonstrates its long-term commitment to people with asthma by encouraging the implementation of these rights and by including asthma in the Health of the Nation strategy.

Published by permission of the National Asthma Campaign.

Index